Creative Bodies in Thera
Performance and Comm

Creative Bodies in Therapy, Performance and Community champions several diverse and innovative approaches in the professional engagement with the creative body as a catalyst for change in therapy, education, somatics and performance.

With contributors from the wide-ranging fields of performance and visual arts, psychotherapy, dance and somatics, this book articulates practice-based experiences in a creative language. The readers are invited to move from the process of reading, into the experience of being in and making sense of the world through a moving body. The book meanders purposefully through practice-led embodied approaches in research that generate new knowledge, methodological frameworks that have emerged in response to the needs of different contexts, as well as offering a window on first-hand experience as practice.

The book will appeal to a wide range of practitioners and trainees in Dance Movement Psychotherapy, arts therapies, counselling and psychotherapy, somatics, community practice and performance.

Caroline Frizell, PhD, is senior lecturer and researcher at Goldsmiths, University of London, as well as therapist and supervisor working indoors and out. She is committed to posthuman, eco-feminist perspectives, working at the intersections of Dance Movement Psychotherapy, ecopsychotherapy and critical disability studies.

Marina Rova, PhD, is programme convenor, lecturer and researcher at Goldsmiths, University of London and co-founder of Arts Minded CIC. Her work is nourished by embodied and relational approaches to knowing and being-in-the-world and led by a curiosity about the developmental, existential and socio-political contexts that shape our narratives.

Creative Bodies in Therapy, Performance and Community

Research and Practice that Brings Us Home

Edited by
Caroline Frizell and Marina Rova

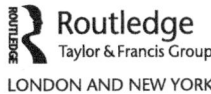

LONDON AND NEW YORK

Cover image: Yannis Kapsaskis

First published 2023
by Routledge
4 Park Square, Milton Park, Abingdon, Oxon OX14 4RN

and by Routledge
605 Third Avenue, New York, NY 10158

Routledge is an imprint of the Taylor & Francis Group, an informa business

© 2023 selection and editorial matter, Caroline Frizell and
Marina Rova; individual chapters, the contributors

British Library Cataloguing-in-Publication Data
A catalogue record for this book is available from the British Library

Library of Congress Cataloging-in-Publication Data
Names: Frizell, Caroline, editor. | Rova, Marina, editor.
Title: Creative bodies in therapy, performance and community:
research and practice that brings us home / edited by Caroline
Frizell and Marina Rova.
Description: Abingdon; New York, NY: Routledge, 2023. |
Includes bibliographical references and index.
Identifiers: LCCN 2022028200 (print) | LCCN 2022028201 (ebook) |
ISBN 9781032119809 (paperback) | ISBN 9781032119816 (hardcover) |
ISBN 9781003222484 (ebook)
Subjects: LCSH: Creative ability—Research.
Classification: LCC BF408 .C6924 2023 (print) |
LCC BF408 (ebook) | DDC 153.3/5—dc23/eng/20221017
LC record available at https://lccn.loc.gov/2022028200
LC ebook record available at https://lccn.loc.gov/2022028201

ISBN: 9781032119816 (hbk)
ISBN: 9781032119809 (pbk)
ISBN: 9781003222484 (ebk)

DOI: 10.4324/9781003222484

Typeset in Bembo
by codeMantra

Contents

Figures

Acknowledgements

We acknowledge, with gratitude, the authors who have contributed to this book. We have been inspired by each and everyone of you, as representatives of a professional field of dance and somatic practitioners, and we thank you for your commitment and unique contribution in this project. We also acknowledge the people whose stories inform the writing of these chapters as well as the animals, places and spaces that have influenced the authors. With thanks also to the technology that has allowed this process to come into being and the materiality of the more-than-human world that has enabled us, as editors, to complete this task. We would like to thank Dr Jill Westwood specifically for providing a creative Foreword for this anthology, the many other colleagues at Goldsmiths, University of London who have inspired each of us in different ways and Yannis Kapsaskis for allowing us to use his artwork.

We both acknowledge those who we love and who love us (human and more than human): without their support this anthology would not have been possible.

Contributors

Archana Ballal

Archana is a UK-based Dance Movement Psychotherapist who has worked with survivors of sexual violence, in the prison sector and youth offending, with Looked After Children/Care Leavers; and in higher education with students in professional dance training. Archana has a background of professional dance performance, choreography and teaching.

Goretti Barjacoba-Souto

Goretti Barjacoba-Souto is a UK registered Dance Movement Psychotherapist (DMP) working with children and young adults with profound and multiple learning disabilities, autism and learning difficulties. She has also experience working with older adults, in main-stream schools and adult mental health, including some research studies for the National Health Service.

Dawn Batcup

Dawn Batcup is a Goldsmiths University Lecturer, Medium Secure Unit Psychotherapist and clinical supervisor part time. Coming from General and Psychiatric Nurse trainings with a Human sciences degree, she has worked in the NHS for almost 40 years, qualifying also as a DMP, Mentalization-Based Therapy (MBT), Group Work and Systemic Practitioner.

Paul Beaumont

Paul is a Registered Somatic Movement Therapist (ISMETA), supervisor and teacher with 20 years' experience working with the body and movement. He is on the faculty of the Institute of Integrative Bodywork & Movement Therapy and works with people of all ages in private practice and with adopted children and families.

Marrianne Behm

Marrianne Behm is an Arts Psychotherapist with over 20 years' experience in NHS clinical settings and also has a private practice in London for supervision and personal therapy. She is a lecturer on the IATE Integrative

Arts Psychotherapy MA course. Marrianne combines a psychodynamic approach with integrative arts models.

Sarah Black-Frizell

Dr Sarah Black-Frizell is course leader for dance at Liverpool Hope University specialising in situated dance, installation practices, maternal and feminist ethics in performance, choreographic methodologies. Sarah works with her composer husband Andy Frizell, her two children on developing a performance practice situated in their family home – *Mother as Curator.*

Claire Burrell

Claire is a Dance Movement Psychotherapist (RDMP, ADMPUK), supervisor and artist taking dance improvisation into cross-modal and transdisciplinary practices with filmmakers, photographers and arts therapists. Claire's clinical practice covers NHS adult mental health and refugee services. She is co-founder of ArtsMinded CIC and visiting lecturer on DMP MA programmes.

Juliet Diener

Juliet is founder and CEO of icandance, a Dance Movement Psychotherapist (ADMPUK and UKCP), supervisor, inclusive dance specialist, trained ballet teacher and educator. Juliet integrates her expertise in education, dance and psychotherapeutic approaches to lead and research creative, inclusive communities. Juliet is currently a Doctoral candidate, researching the work of icandance.

Ditty Doktor

Dr Ditty Dokter, FPC, UKCP, HCPC, BADth, ADMPUK, was course leader in MA Dramatherapy at Anglia Ruskin University, Cambridge until 2016 and continues to offer therapy, teaching and clinical supervision in private practice. She is an internationally renowned researcher and author, having published widely in the field of the arts therapies.

Caroline Frizell

Caroline is senior lecturer on MA Dance Movement Psychotherapy at Goldsmiths, which she convened from 2010 to 2019. Caroline holds a PhD in posthuman, eco-feminist research and practises in psychotherapy and supervision (UKCP, ADMP), including environmental outdoor work. Caroline's extensive publications intersect DMP, ecopsychotherapy, supervision and critical disability studies.

Agnes Law

Agnes has been a registered private practitioner and supervisor (ADMPUK) since 2013. She is a lecturer on the MA Dance Movement Psychotherapy at Goldsmiths, faculty member of School of Playback Theatre, UK and founding member of True Heart Theatre. Her areas of interest include reflective practice, learning through action and intersectionality.

Heidrun Panhofer

Heidrun is associate professor in the Department of Clinical Psychology at the Autonomous University in Barcelona. She has been directing the Master's Programme in DMT since 2003. Her research covers the fields of DMT teaching and supervision, the embodied mind, interculturality, attachment, different client populations and movement observation and analysis.

Angela Pierre Louis

Angie lectures at Liverpool Hope University. Her interests lie in widening participation through facilitation improvisation, dance making, performance, contemporary technique, which is somatically informed.

Helen Poynor

Helen Poynor runs the ***Walk of Life*** Training and Workshop Programme in Non-stylised and Environmental Movement. An RDMP & RSMT trained intensively with Anna Halprin and Suprapto Suryodarmo, she mentors practitioners and publishes widely. An independent movement artist, Helen specialises in movement in natural environments, site-specific/autobiographical performance and artistic collaborations.

Marina Rova

Marina is programme convenor, lecturer and researcher (Goldsmiths University of London) and co-founder of Arts Minded CIC. Marina's professional background includes clinical practice in adult NHS mental health settings, perinatal psychiatry and dementia services and independent consultancy work for charitable organisations. She holds an interdisciplinary PhD on Kinaesthetic Empathy (2017).

Ellen Steinmüller

Ellen Steinmüller is a professionally trained contemporary dancer, experienced Community Dance Artist and qualified Dance Movement Psychotherapist with substantial clinical practice. With over 15 years of professional experience, her practice is focused on effecting processes of social empowerment and personal transformation. Ellen is a Doctoral student at Ludwig-Maximilians-University Munich, Germany.

Jill Westwood

Jill Westwood, PhD, is an artist-art psychotherapist-researcher, programme convenor MA Art Psychotherapy at Goldsmiths University (2009–2020) and Course Advisor MA Art Therapy and Graduate Diploma in Expressive Therapies at Western Sydney University, Australia (1995–2007). Her publications include co-editorship of *Art Therapy in Australia: Taking a Postcolonial, Aesthetic Turn*. Brill Sense (2019).

Foreword

Dr. Jill Westwood

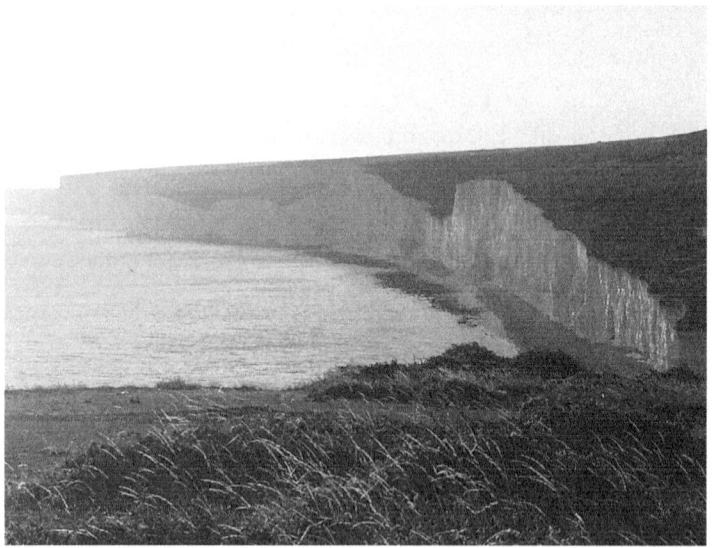

Figure i Seven Sisters. Jill Westwood, digital photograph (2018).

This book invites you into your body, the rhythm of your breath, the experience of your senses. Prepare to be taken on a profound and tender dance through these pages. As you step through this discursive, wild garden, assemblage. Taking a cliff path facing the sea, to meet the agency of your own performance in a catalyst for change.

Its contents will call you to join a community of authors who locate creative process at the heart of their embodied participatory practices. And, to immerse yourself in dancing together as their experiences become entangled with your own as you move through and bear witness to their contributions, touching the painful, compassionate, emancipatory material of this work. You will travel inside institutions such as hospitals, prisons and into homes, communities and countries to meet people participating in this interconnected group-dance to find empathic resonance and profound transformation. Everybody is included in this community-making towards dismantling structures of oppression.

In response to this anthology, I began with an image (Figure i). A photograph of the "Seven Sisters" taken on one of many occasional walks, along the path of this iconic and liminal site. On this day, the beach was closed and empty of people due to a rock fall. An undulating, prehistoric, lime-stone-chalk, cliff edge embedded with bands of tabular flint; it is home to countless flora, fauna, human settlement, and defences over millennia, and an image of British "homeland". It is a place where the cliff gradually and inexorably crumbles into the sea.

This is a place of intra-action, of friendships, sisterhood, art activities and memories. Of sleeping out the night of a summer solstice in the 1980s with friends, lighting a fire and wrapping our bodies in a sheet of polythene as protection from the drizzling rain as we lay on the hard pebbles. Of swimming naked in cool sparkling waters on warm summer days of birthday celebrations. A place of a guided, art-based, silent walk during early Spring; encountering the wonder of a snakelet on the path. Of walking with friends and dogs in bracing Winter winds and driving rain while collecting materials of hag stones, seaweeds and crow feathers to make into a hybrid creature; in the form of human-female-crow-donkey pregnant and in a state of pupation (Figure ii). She became a crucible of imagination, gestating complex emotional associations and a coalescence of my role as an artist-art psychotherapist-educator-researcher that stood in watch in various sites, exhibitions and in my work-grotto for many years. A form subsequently, ritualistically dissolved when I left my post at Goldsmiths and given back to the earth as compost (Figure iii). Simultaneously giving birth to a baby named "Pan" into the care of trusted colleagues (Figure iv). This diffraction recognises a dynamism of forces where everything is interconnected and entangled. Moving us towards a place where things cannot be separated from each other. This inspired book of dance research and practice is significant in this quest, and in bringing us home into our creative bodies and moving us towards changing the way we participate in knowing, becoming and seeking questions we are not yet aware of.

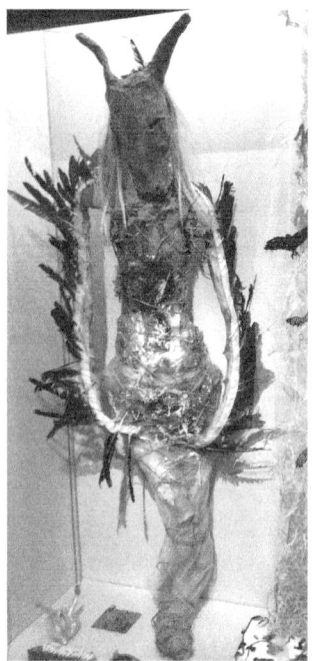

Figure ii Hybrid Creature. Jill Westwood, Digital Photograph (2015).

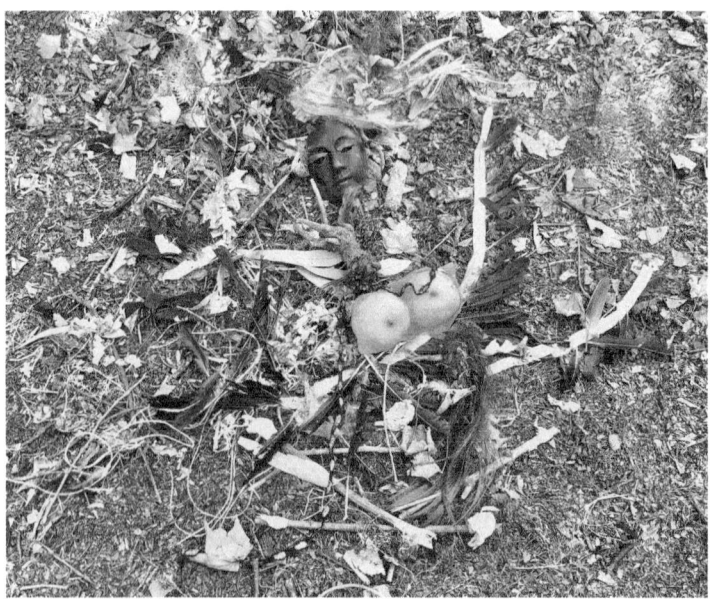

Figure iii Dissolving into the Earth. Jill Westwood, digital photograph (2020).

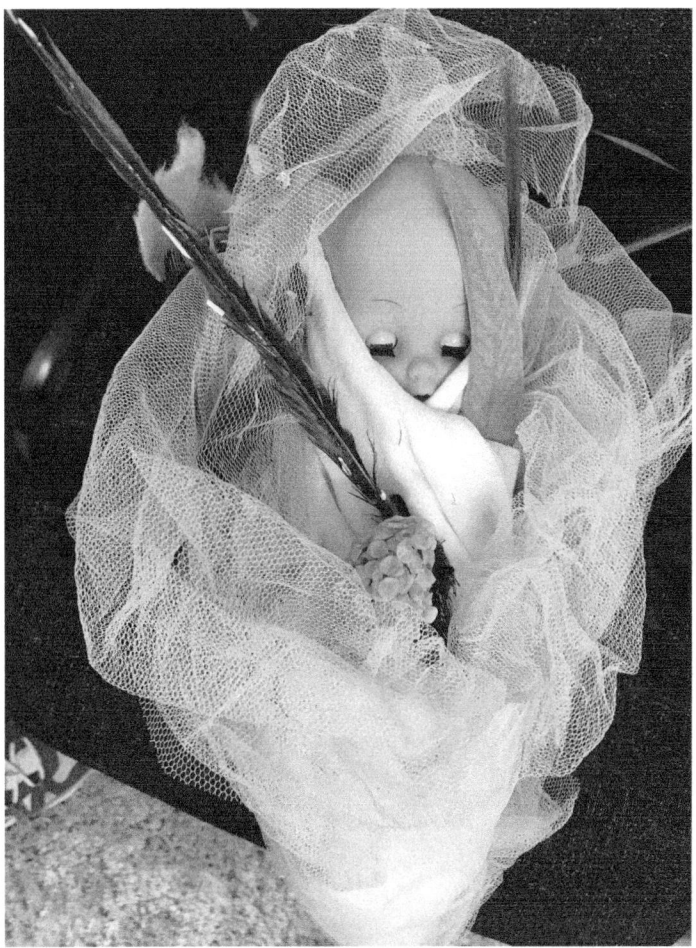

Figure iv Baby Pan. Jill Westwood, digital photograph (2020).

1 Arriving, becoming and arriving again

Caroline Frizell and Marina Rova

In editing this anthology of works, we have welcomed embodied creativity into the heart of innovative research, methodological frameworks for practice and practice-in-its-very-becoming. The anthology spans a palette of colour, beginning with approaches in research that identify how embodied practice itself generates new knowledge. These approaches include phenomenology, new materialism, arts-based research and case study. We then invite you into chapters that explore the different theoretical scaffoldings that have emerged in response to the needs of different contexts, such as children and young people with disabilities, care leavers, forensics and hard-to-reach populations working on the interface of dance as therapy, as performance and as a community practice. The final chapters then offer a window on practice as a first-hand experience, centring moment-to-moment experiences in the primacy of the moving body. The contributors represent a wide lineage, with professional identities that span multiple sources, from mother-artists, to community dance artists, to performers, to somatic therapists to arts psychotherapists. Their research and practice includes non-stylised movement, improvisational dance and dance as participation in the world. This book aims to develop discourses and theorise embodied practice. In doing so, we wish to challenge assumptions about the ways we can work with our creative bodies and also about the ways we articulate the process itself. This returns us to a child-like wonder as illustrated spontaneously by four-year old Yannis in Figure 1.1.

The idea for this project gathered momentum at a professional junction of the two women editors of this book, Caroline and Marina. The setting for this junction was academia; specifically, the Dance Movement Psychotherapy (DMP) MA at Goldsmiths, University of London. On arriving at this junction, Caroline was a research-active senior lecturer, who had worked on the programme for 15 years and was seeking to step away from ten years of the administrative demands of the role of programme convenor. This way she could devote more time to developing research. Caroline considered herself an academic migrant. She entered academia after many years of combining community dance practice alongside family caring roles and motherhood that included mothering a learning-disabled, now adult daughter. She

DOI: 10.4324/9781003222484-1

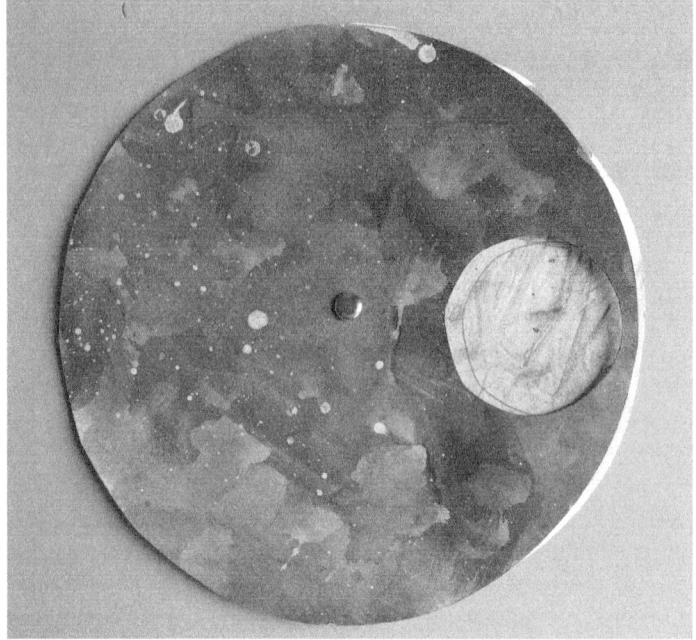

Figure 1.1 The Universe. Artwork by Yannis Kapsaskis, age four years.

considered that, at this junction, she might even finish that PhD that had been on the back burner for so many years. Marina was entering Goldsmiths as a research-active lecturer, stepping into the staff team as programme convenor, having completed her PhD some years earlier and now eager to find an arena in which she could further her academic curiosity. Before migrating to Goldsmiths, Marina had spent 15 years at another academic institution (University of Roehampton), her first academic home, initially as a student and later as a lecturer and researcher. The two women were a generation apart: Caroline in her sixties with three grown-up daughters and Marina on the cusp of her forties, with a young son. Both came into DMP via ballet school and subsequent professional dance training and both were (are) steeped in, and committed to movement, dance and creativity as the mainstay of the (post)human experience. We both subscribe to eco-feminist principles of the ethics of care, compassion and kindness, as well as defiance, resilience and resistance in the face of patriarchal oppression and in the name of social justice.

This book emerged in the 21st-century, post-colonial turn and the meeting place for this collaboration was the context of Higher Education, which itself was groaning under the vicissitudes of neoliberal agendas hellbent on the marketisation of education, like woodworm devouring the integrity of critical pedagogy. Our initial ideas for this book were about bringing together embodied research, practice and scholarship, always within the orbit of creativity. At the same time, we were finding that Higher Education was becoming increasingly managerial and we found ourselves swimming against the tide. The union were calling strikes in the name of equality and justice for the university community, and our conversations continued on the picket lines. Just as the strikes were coming to an end, the pandemic burst into the public arena and we found ourselves in lockdown, needing to navigate our processes as researchers, practitioners and educators, who valued the kinaesthetic wisdom of the material body, through a screen. This was a new world.

Caroline, a Celtic-native (identifying for the majority of her life as a North Londoner) of the land in which our paths met. Marina an EU immigrant arriving in the UK from Greece in 2002. Perhaps not uncommon for a migrant, place, space and belonging have always occupied Marina's world. Where IS home, truly, for a cultural nomad? In conversation, we discovered that as writers we both identify as academic migrants. Caroline's arrival into formal academia later in life after years of activism and DMP practice and Marina's working-class background and acquisition of academic English, as an adult, remind us that class, language, geographical location, socio-political context, age, ability, gender, race, ethnicity and care responsibilities intersect and shape not only our experience-in-the-world but also our trajectories in life (Crenshaw 1989).

Having met obliquely in passing on their way through the professional field of DMP, Caroline and Marina met in person at Goldsmiths as Marina began her work there. As practitioners, we arrive, again and again, into our practice. The demand for continued professional development brings our attention to this sense of fluidity as we move through what we know and allow it to be affected, interrupted and transformed, again and again. Heidrun Panhoffer (Chapter 2) explores the process of checking in. Arrival is really important: sometimes just to arrive is enough; just to pitch up; to be present. All matter arrives somehow into this world and that is its gift; that it is here. There is a playful ambiguity in the idea of arrival, in that it is also simultaneously a departure.

Marina sent Caroline a text:

'just arrived'.

She had wandered down the long chequered corridor to arrive at the café. Marina could feel a knot in her stomach as she waited for Caroline's arrival. The warmth of the paper cup, filled to the brim with black coffee, held between the palms of her hands soothed her nervous anticipation about the transition she was making. This reminded her of landing. Will her landing be smooth or bumpy? Will her new environment be welcoming or hostile? Would she meet a kindred spirit in Caroline's face?

Caroline responded to the text:

'...meet you in the café in five minutes...'

Caroline was sitting in her office, immersed in the never-ending programme convenor's to-do list that she would be keen to hand over. She straightened her spine and pushed her elbows backwards to open her chest. Sitting in her black swivel chair, she twisted her body with arms outstretched, catching sight of the hand-written poem on the wall entitled 'A short story of falling' (Oswald 2016). This had been a poem that she had used in the introductory workshop to welcome a fresh cohort of students into the new academic year. It was written in her best handwriting and blu-tacked to her office wall. She lingered on the first two lines:

> '…It is the story of the falling rain
> to turn into a leaf and fall again…'

(1)

The words conjured the image of a tiny raindrop, suspended in the air as it descended towards the leaf, to slide down that shiny green surface in slow motion, before continuing its fall. The poem on the wall seemed a hundred miles away from the spreadsheet on the computer screen with which she had been struggling. It was a reminder of the creativity that falls continuously through her body, chancing upon a leaf before it continues through the channel of infinity. She took a breath and stood up. There was a bubble of excitement in her stomach, quivering like the surface tension of the raindrop at the prospect of this new meeting point. That image of the raindrop in its falling towards the leaf hung as an embodied turning point in which our material presence in the world is always imbued with our affective capacity. This place of embodied presence is so central to the chapters in this book. For example, in Chapter 8, 'Breath, Belly and Back. Dropping into Body as Ground,' Paul Beaumont writes so eloquently about the creative potential that is held within the aliveness of the body. Helen Poynor (Chapter 9) illustrates how the body knows what needs to be expressed, if only we can allow it to have a voice, in her chapter entitled 'Is that yoga or are you just making it up?'.

Both Caroline and Marina have contributed single-authored chapters about the place of embodied knowing in research. In her chapter 'Kinaesthetic entanglements and creative immersion in embodied performance', Marina Rova (Chapter 4) takes us into the visceral experience of everyday life enactments that touch powerful emotions as relational dramas unfold. She then goes on to explore research, drawing parallels between the way in which creativity and performance provide a catalyst from which insights can emerge in relation to wider issues about how we affect and are affected by each other in a rapidly changing world. Marina argues that we can nurture compassionate qualities through building increasing embodied awareness. We shift between performer and audience and together they create an inter-dependent narrative. The research moves away from the binary of (active/doing) performer and (passive/receiving) audience, to a more mutual doing-together of this performance thing. Caroline Frizell's pathbreaking research discussed in 'The cat, the foal and other meetings that make a difference: posthuman research that re-animates our responsiveness to knowing and becoming' (Chapter 5) unpacks the materiality of moving relational bodies as our intra-active posthuman subjectivity and ground for knowing-in-the-world. Caroline's work challenges normative assumptions about what constitutes research but also what it means to be human. Care and eco-ethical research and practice are at the heart of Caroline's writing. Through weaving critical disability theory, eco-psychotherapy, embodied practice, and conscious and less-conscious experiences of the everyday, Caroline asks us to consider the ways in which we can explore how embodied creativity changes the way we participate in the world.

Moving back to Alice Oswald's (2016) poem, handwritten on what was then Caroline's office wall (and is now Marina's office), she asks:

'…if only I a passerby could pass
as clear as water through a plume of grass
to find the sunlight hidden at the tip
turning to seed a kind of lifting rain drip…'

It is these transient moments of potential that infuse this book with the process of becoming through the primacy of the moving body, always moving towards meeting points that bring the potential for new ways to experience the world. As Caroline and Marina met in that café a connection was made, as a raindrop meets a leaf.

This meeting was at a particular social junction in time, as inequalities and oppressions were awakening the sleeping beauties of public awareness. Terrible violence and injustices that had become normalised were now being publicly challenged. For example, George Floyd's murder by a white police officer galvanised the Black Lives Matter movement, as individual and institutional racism that had oppressed so many lives over centuries became unveiled in the public arena. As this chapter is being written, anti-racism campaigners have been cleared for toppling the statue of a slave trader in Bristol. The UK faces up to its colonial past. The #Metoo movement was giving women a voice to call out sexual violence and refuse the misogyny that had become common currency. The environmental crisis could no longer be ignored, as floods, wildfires and plastic in the ocean threatened (not just human) lives and shocked the world. This writing comes in the wake of a splintering Brexit campaign, which began in 2016 and the UK finally left the European Union in 2020, at once destabilising EU nationals living in the UK and UK nationals living in the EU. A divisive 'them and us' discourse was cultivated by the UK government, who promised to 'make Britain great again' by tackling migration and taking back control of policy making and trade deals. And in the process of this book coming into fruition, there are scandalous revelations that those in power, who, at the same time as demanding restrictions of the public in the pandemic that meant folk were left to die alone and to mourn alone, were holding 'bring your own booze parties' in the gardens of number ten Downing Street.

Injustice is rife and the seeds of this book were sown in the crisis of the Covid-19 pandemic. The pandemic disrupted ways of living and as embodied practitioners, educators and researchers, we found that our professional practices, in which socio-kinetic exchanges were so crucial, moved our work into online screens. Throughout the book, you will find references to how embodied practitioners, educators and researchers navigated the pandemic and its implications for working with movement.

Ideas and practices of social justice are woven through the book. For example, Archana Ballal's chapter 'Dancing in the Kitchen: Using Creativity and Embodiment to Promote a Decolonising Approach to Psychotherapy' (Chapter 12) asks you, the reader, to challenge the assumptions and codes of practice that support the work of therapists and to question established practices that have been colonised by cultural norms. In a similar vein, Ellen Steinmüller (Chapter 7) brings us her work with Dance United, illustrating how dance performance can empower young people with mental health issues in 'Lives transformed through dance: the art of dance as a catalyst for personal transformation'. These are just two of several chapters that illustrate how dance and movement practices can bring about social change. This theme of social justice weaves colourful threads throughout the book and in her chapter 'Finding my way home: an embodied journey to building an inclusive dance community' Juliet Diener (Chapter 11) demonstrates how working on the interfaces of dance as therapy, performance and community practice can foster communities that welcome children and young people with disabilities and their families, providing them with a sense of belonging in a world that can be experienced as hostile by those who defy normative assumptions. This theme of social justice widens out into issues of migration that can be found echoed in Ditty Dokter's chapter 'Arts based research and self-reflexive autobiographical performance' (Chapter 3), in which performance work becomes a way of making sense of the unique individual experience of being othered, in relation to wider discourses of migration. This theme becomes threaded through other chapters, such as Claire Burrell's 'Being Seen and Seeing Self: Explorations in the Creative Process in Performance and Therapy' (Chapter 10) where the author asks us to consider the ways in which we frame, make visible and witness embodiment and how this process informs how we view ourselves and others.

In the structure of the book, the focal points sometimes emerge as distinct from each other, such as in the articulation of research practices, the methodological scaffolding that informs practice or the first-hand experience of the practice itself. But more often, these strands become entangled in the richness of the work, such as when the practice is the research and when the research is the practice. The contributing chapters are sequenced to offer an assemblage that moves through, and questions permeable boundaries, challenging and developing the discourses that exist in relation to dance and somatic practices and research. This book is about arriving back home into the materiality of the body.

As individuals and professionals, we (Caroline and Marina) write with an understanding of being an outsider. At the same time, we recognise our privilege in having the opportunity to collaborate and co-edit this anthology. We wonder about the conflict arising from being an outsider and having a platform at the same time. Perhaps, it is not a conflict as such but more accurately, it is a responsibility we have as editors and writers, to speak with integrity about these outsider experiences. This is illustrated by the stories unfolding in the pages of this book. The stories of outsiders such as care leavers, learning disabled people, adults living with a mental illness, incarcerated individuals, patients in forensic services and people with refugee status. All the chapters in this anthology grapple with different ways that we (as practitioners and individuals) can foster connection, integration and growth, often in the midst of adversity or during challenging phases in our life span.

The idea of this edited anthology emerged from a desire to bring together a community of authors who could bring their embodied practice from the studio and outdoor spaces into the written word. At the beginning of this project, we wanted to become clearer about the direction of this book and by chance, we had attended a writing workshop held as staff development at Goldsmiths with Dr Diedre Daley, a lecturer in academic literacies. Both of us, Caroline and Marina, were inspired by the simplicity of this workshop, in which small provocations got the creative juices flowing. The sometimes overwhelming task of producing meaningful text became a joy and an intrigue. Following this, we committed to a couple of hours in a studio to allow the project of this anthology to germinate, with some coloured pens and large pieces of paper and offered each other small provocations, to which we responded in turn through movement and then let the pens write or draw as seemed fit while the other witnessed. The process was creative and productive, and a focus for the yet-to-be created book became clearer in terms of the creative moving body serving a resource to enable each of us to become more present to our affective capacity as part of the wider world. The challenge of this book was to present research, methodology and practice in a way that reflects the experiential, immersive and emergent character of the practice itself.

Embodied creativity was (is) where we feel at home and the process through which each author has nourished their practice and personal development. As the term anthology denotes, and much like a flower, each chapter was borne out of a specific ecosystem, cultivated in its own soil and nourished within diverse climes and environments. We invited authors who were from different professional and academic traditions. Though they are all experienced practitioners, some are mature writers in their respective fields while others are beginning to take their first steps as authors. Taken together the chapters in this collection create a metaphor for multiplicity and possibility arising at the intersections of dance, somatic and therapy practice. Put simply, this book is about making connections, staying connected and playing with the transformation of knowing between modalities.

Collaborative thinking permeated the process of editing this book. We created meeting opportunities on Zoom, either in groups or individually, where authors shared their writing process, sometimes through painful exploration. As editors we had to navigate the tension arising between our commitment to develop thematic congruence for the book and allowing freedom for authors to bring their own voice to the writing. We hope that these negotiations were handled with care. We acknowledge the authors who began with us and later chose to step away from this project. We hope that the seeds of their writing will continue to grow elsewhere. The writing process opened up stimulating conversations among authors about allowing ourselves to be vulnerable, the notion of intra-active choice and finding fluidity in being with what emerges. The actual becoming of the book then echoes its core premise: foregrounding creative bodies as practice is a catalyst for change.

Though this book is predominantly written by female authors, this is not a homogenous female voice. Some of the chapters concern themselves with women's work specifically. Sarah and Angie (Chapter 6) share their *Offerings* with us. The chapter is itself an event that straddles performance, relationship, social commentary and research inquiry through sited dance practice, improvisation, ethics and the maternal. The pandemic amplified personal/professional entanglements as families found their routines severely disrupted in terms of work, school, domestic duties and childcare. Sarah and Angie demonstrate how their chapter '*Offerings* tells the stories of our lives in movement' is about giving and receiving with ethical care and with sensitivity. They create art work together that arises out of turbulent times. This art work creates an historical statement about a particular kind of embodied feminism that is exposed in the exceptional circumstance of the pandemic.

Experiences of motherhood and female identity are handed down from one generation to the next. Agnes Law refers to her grandmother's beginnings as a formative anti-oppressive narrative informing her own process of becoming and her work with incarcerated women years later. Agnes's chapter 'Sing your way home: Designing a creative group intervention in the women's prison as a Dance Movement Therapist in Singapore' (Chapter 13) brings Playback theatre into the arena, a process in which performers and audience are mutually implicated in what is created. Here, a community theatre practice is transported into a female prison and acts as a bridge during the women's transition and re-integration in society. In 'Borderlands: Exploring creativity as a practice of liminality in the arts therapies' (Chapter 14), Marina Rova and Marrianne Behm delve into four women's experiences of living with depression. The authors invite us into the liminal and transformative space of creativity as they deconstruct embodied practice through the process of movement improvisation and art making, utilised in a mixed-modality arts therapy group.

Other female authors write about work with male clients. Dawn Batcup's powerful account of 'Indominus Rex; developing mentalisation with offenders through externalisation and creativity in a Dance Movement Psychotherapy

Group' (Chapter 15) reveals the complexity of working therapeutically with extremely distressed clients in a forensic setting. Dawn integrates creativity, mentalisation and psychodynamic process to support the therapeutic relationship and reveals the importance of connection (with disparate parts of ourselves) and integration (physical, mental and emotional) towards recovery and change. Goretti Barjacoba-Souto's moving chapter, written in letter form, 'Dancing with Stephen: Reconnecting with the Body in a Search for Closure' (Chapter 16) speaks of the unbearable loss of a child client and explores embodied creativity as a way of processing and moving through this pain.

Paul Beaumont is the only male voice in this anthology. His chapter 'Breath, Belly and Back. Dropping into Body as Ground' (Chapter 8) offers an alternative narrative to patriarchal views of masculinity as he invites us to consider the multiple ways of knowing by dropping into the body as the ground for our experiences in the world. Paul presents small but profound, political and personal acts of holding spaces for bodies, reminding us that overreliance on verbal or cognitive processing can move us into a disconnection from our material body-in-the-world. Of course, speaking is a bodily act; however, prescribed codes, symbols and conventions assigned to linguistic practices can only go so far when it comes to accessing the breadth and depth of our experiential knowledge.

Can we ever escape the limitations of verbal language in articulating embodied experience? This becomes more complicated in multilingual contexts. As a bilingual speaker, Marina is acutely aware of the linguistic limitations and affordances embedded in different languages. Often, certain words, states or feelings will not translate directly in another language. For example, through her personal linguistic practices interweaving Greek (mother tongue/private language) and English (academic/professional language), she has come to realise that she tends to express affective experiences more fully in her mother tongue (Greek), whereas she tends to process cognitive or analytical thinking more confidently in English. Marina remembers struggling to put her feelings into words as a patient in a London hospital once, feeling so overwhelmed by the experience that the only words she could access were in Greek; unfortunately, this seemed to be of no use in her communication with the impatient doctor carrying out the assessment. We are reminded here of the countless times we have tried to communicate with patients, clients or residents in different therapeutic contexts when *language* is more than just the specific words that we use. Or the times when, in a social context, an inside joke has gone unnoticed because a key cultural reference is missing. With the global movement of populations across borders and countries (linguistic), identity becomes malleable, for example in articulating affective experiences within foreign or unfamiliar cultural contexts. A few authors cross these linguistic and cultural borders through their writing and practice in this book and this is specifically articulated in Ditty Dokter's chapter (Chapter 3) 'Arts based research and self-reflexive autobiographical performance' in which she invites us into the intersections of ageing, disabled and migrant identities.

But spoken or written words are not the only languages that we have. Barad (2003) calls out the way language has been privileged at the expense of the materiality of the world. She says;

> Language has been granted too much power. The linguistic turn, the semiotic turn, the interpretative turn, the cultural turn: it seems that at every turn lately every "thing"—even materiality—is turned into a matter of language or some other form of cultural representation…
>
> (801)

This anthology foregrounds how creativity and corporeality can bring us into new ways of languaging the world. This shift away from the linguistic, semiotic, interpretive and cultural turns manifests strongly in Goretti Barjacoba-Souto's writing (Chapter 16) in which she mourns the death of a young client, Stephen, who had profound and complex needs. Goretti describes the multi-dimensionality of touch as a form of deep connection and communication against all the odds. Similarly, Helen's chapter 'Is that Yoga or are you just making it up' (Chapter 9) reminds us not only that movement is language but the importance of not translating movement into (verbal) language. There is common ground, though this is not neutral or universal, in our (post)human, mortal, moving and relational bodies. This is our capacity to express, communicate and navigate relationships in (and with) the world kinetically and kinaesthetically. This experience is also described as presence (Chapter 8) through Paul's written vignettes and somatic experiencing provocations. Similarly, in 'The Matriarch and the Mollusc' (Chapter 17), Caroline and Helen invite us to attend to our embodied knowing-in-the-world and connection with the more than human. Furthermore, the authors invite us to look beyond our own (kine)sphere and recognise our intra-action with the world and the more than human.

This leaning into the world requires that we are partial to *just making it up* (see Poynor, Chapter 9) in our responsiveness in any one moment. This is the place of improvisation. When we translate embodied experience into language, it becomes something else. Sometimes, the meaning is in the materiality of the experience; in staying with this materiality. Sometimes, poetic language or representation through an art object helps us get closer to what it is we seek. Sometimes, we need to step back and engage with language and discourse to create a conceptualisation. Claire Burrell's exploration (Chapter 10) considers the different ways we can engage with creativity, sometimes to come closer and sometimes to gain a wider perspective into our personal narrative and experience.

Even though the creative moving body is the through line of this book, it is by no means taken for granted as a fixed or definitive practice. As many authors demonstrate in the pages of this anthology, this corporeal turn is not only an intentional attitudinal stance, but it becomes an act of defiance or intervention or a paradigm shift. These activist approaches offer an active engagement with performativity on social, cultural and political levels. The book encourages you, the reader, the opportunity to delve into your own embodied present and embrace your creative moving body in practice and everyday life as a catalyst for change.

Conclusion

This book seeks to challenge the hierarchies of power, questioning how we locate, embody and respond to authority, bringing into focus the nuances embedded in embodied knowledge whilst holding a wider picture in mind. We have sought out contributors from different disciplines, perspectives, backgrounds and geographical locations, all of whom celebrate dance as a life force and all of whom are pioneers in their own way. The book models creativity as practice and research; we are not only writing about it (doing it) but we are living it ourselves (being it) as authors and practitioners. We hope that in reading this book the creative moving body will speak to you as a resource that can enable each of us to become part of the wider world. We have aimed to curate an anthology of works that are accessible not just for practitioners in related fields, but also for the wider public. We have seen communities turn to expressive means of communication through the arts to process trauma, crises and loss. Movement traverses boundaries, borders and cultural differences and has the capacity to hold shared values of our humanity within the broader ecology of the world.

As you navigate the chapters of this book, whether in the linear order it is presented, or through weaving back and forth as your interest takes you, we ask you to attend to your active role of listener, that is, the one who holds the space and enters into a place of witnessing the ideas that emerge.

References

Barad, K. (2003). Posthuman performativity: Matter comes to matter. *Signs: Journal of Women in Culture and Society*, 28 (3), pp. 801–831.

Crenshaw, K. (1989). Demarginalizing the intersection of race and sex: A black feminist critique of antidiscrimination doctrine. *Feminist Theory and Antiracist Politics, University of Chicago Legal Forum*, 140, pp. 139–167.

Oswald, A. (2016). *Falling awake*. London: Penguin Random House.

2 Check-in, please! Exploring movement check-ins as a tool for embodied psychotherapeutic practice

Heidrun Panhofer

Beginnings

A typical setting of Dance Movement Therapy (DMT) sessions initiates with a check-in, a space which allows participants to take conscience and share how they are feeling, both physically and emotionally (Curtis 2002; Meekums 2002; Panhofer & Rodríguez Cigaran 2005). The idea is, just like on a journey, to check-in one's baggage before getting on to a plane, to ensure maximum mobility and freedom for the traveller. But it also allows both the client and the therapist to learn more about the expectations and burdens for this common expedition.

Different approaches of how to conduct this initial check-in have been described, using art, movement or verbal sharing (e.g., Dietrich-Hartwell et al. 2020; Meekums 2002, 2008; Savidaki et al. 2020; Valdivia 2010). The therapist is supposed to take on the client's luggage or, viewed through psychoanalytic lenses, the client's projections in order to contain these and carry along a piece of the shared journey. A dance movement therapist also uses her/his/their skills of movement observation and analysis to become aware of any nonverbal cues that might help to understand the clients' inner world (Denham & Onwuegbuzie 2013; Moore & Yamamoto 2011; Payne 2017), in particular for those client groups who have a hard time connecting with their emotional or physical states. Verbalising what is happening in one's inner world is quite challenging for many (Panhofer 2011), and this can be even harder in middle- or large-sized groups[1] (Panhofer et al. 2014).

Given these circumstances, a specific movement check-in has been created at our training programme in DMT at the Autonomous University in Barcelona. Identifying with different shades of states, it facilitates participants to connect psychophysically with their emotional and physical states of being. Bridging the bodily and emotional experience, the nonverbal and verbal, the movement check-in proposes an active exploration and sharing in movement. Groups with a higher level of anxiety or dependence, such as at the beginning when members are not familiar yet with each other, the space and the activity, may need more direction: For example, participants may be asked directly to embody the amount of vitality they have right now, situating themselves anywhere between down

DOI: 10.4324/9781003222484-2

on the floor for tiredness and up high close to the ceiling for plenty of vitality. No matter how participants feel, they are invited to choose a certain level in the space, connect with their moving bodies and corporealise their personal energy state. However, the activity remains dynamic at all times, nobody is supposed to remain static on one level; sometimes, one and the same body perceives different states, for example, a tired back may curve downwards while sparkling eyes may explore higher spheres. Sometimes, movement changes one's initial state and after a few stretches close to the ground one's vitality increases, lifting the body to a medium level. Everybody is invited to play and connect with different places within the continuum:

Should the members of the group not know each other, direct questions that are of relevance for this group could be asked to promote familiarity. For example, for a newly composed group with many commuters or travellers, it could be suggested that all those who are at home nearby could locate themselves in the centre of the place. Others, who are commuting or who have just arrived, could move about or locate themselves at the edges of the space. How far am I from home?

> *Who else lives, just like me, in Barcelona? Who is taking a train, bus or plane, to arrive here for the weekend? Who has left his/her/their country and culture and moved here most recently? I watch students of the introductory course, who have met each other for the first time this morning, exchanging empathetic glances as they are invited to get a feeling of the large panorama of the group.*
>
> (*From* the field notes of the researcher)

After an initial time of connecting with one's own necessities, expressing one's personal states and playing with the opposites of the same continuum, the participants are invited to connect with other members and become aware of the larger picture of the group.

> *A pair in the corner discover that each has crossed the Atlantic Ocean to come here and study, getting a grip of each other's forearm. A little group of commuters gathers travelling from the centre to the edge of the space with an energetic step, engaging in a similar rhythm. Even though the journey has not been the same, the different experiences of the participants are somehow acknowledged, and first connections are made.*
>
> (*From* the field notes of the researcher)

Becoming aware of the rest of the group not only represents an important step of situating oneself within the group, but also offers a bridge from a more individual warm-up to an interactive phase of play and exchange.

> *I asked the students to become aware of their emotional states, in particular how anxious or serene they were feeling at this present moment. Those who rather connected with peace and calmness I invited to move less, tending towards stillness while I suggested representing a lot of anxiety with a lot of movement. Students*

experimented with different parts of the body and incorporated different speeds in their movements. Soon it became apparent that a large majority engaged in sustained, almost Thai-Chi-like movements, whereas two participants gradually sped up. Both of the participants had mentioned preoccupations and doubts during the prior short verbal check-in and now started shaking different body parts and restlessly looking around. As their gazes met, they started running with each other, chasing around between a landscape of statue-like peers.

(*From* the field notes of the researcher)

No matter how directive, the movement check-in invites participants to learn to pay attention to themselves, become aware and express their different states, while experiencing the climate of the entire group. As the group advances, it needs less direction and develops its own language and dynamics of attuning with oneself and with others.

This chapter explores movement check-ins, intertwining open-ended questionnaires, a focus group (Bergold & Thomas 2012; Kitzinger 1995), the researcher's field notes, and the existing literature, to further the development of this technique, but also searching to enhance processes of beginnings in therapy.

The proceedings

As a first step, in order to learn more about the movement check-ins, it seemed inevitably to address those who had experienced the technique. An online inquiry with a total of 30 questions was thus created via the platform Survey Monkey Questionnaire, allowing students to evaluate on a Likert-scale their complete agreement or disagreement, but also inviting them to provide further comments and observations. The first ten questions looked at the general utility of the movement check-ins as such: in how far the activity had been helpful to connect with one's own physicality or emotional states, or to what extent it had aided to find one's place in the group, take conscience of the group's climate, to connect with others or to learn about their physical and emotional conditions. The second part of the questionnaire scrutinised the various possibilities of embodying the different states, for example, in how far it had been helpful to embody one's tiredness with movements on a low level in the space, one's anxiety with a lot of movement, or one's connectedness to the group right in the centre of the crowd, or one's well-being with an open body posture. This second part thus aimed to assess the different bodily representations that had been suggested by the facilitator, unexpectedly entering the field of movement observation and analysis. Evaluating bodily communication by an intercultural group stemming from several countries, cultures and continents, as is usual for our university training, seemed somehow a challenging task.

An invitation to participate in the online survey was sent to a total of 60 students from the masters and postgraduate training at the Autonomous University of Barcelona, 42 first- and 18 second-year students, excluding the third-year cohort as their lived experience of the movement check-ins seemed more remote. Forty-five students aged between 24 and 49 and stemming from 14 different countries completed the survey. Seven confirmed their participation in an online focus group, once the results of the survey had been published, out of which six actually were able to attend the one-hour lasting online event.

The Focus Group, an organised discussion with a selected group of individuals to obtain information on the ideas, attitudes and viewpoints around a specific topic (Bergold & Thomas 2012; Kitzinger 1995), centred around three themes that had emerged from the questionnaires, i.e. the possibility to connect to oneself through the movement check-in, the possibility to connect to other members of the group, and the suitability of representing different states through movement. A last space was offered for general comments and suggestions, offering a space for all those comments that had not emerged via the survey and gathering thus a bank of qualitative data alongside the quantitative outcomes of the survey.

The findings I: May movement check-ins be useful?

The outcome of the Survey Monkey assessment showed an extremely high approval of the usefulness of the movement check-ins. Connecting with different associations and representing them physically was thought to be useful by 95% of the participants, in particular in order to recognise one's own physical (41% of the complete agreement, 43% agreement) and emotional states (39% complete agreement, 48% agreement). Participants mentioned that the movement check-in "allowed me to get in touch with improvisation and my corporality, exactly what I needed in that moment", and "I did not know how I felt that day and so I just tried both extremes and moved in between, listening to what felt better in that instant". "It helped me to connect with the present moment", and "I managed to unblock certain repressed sensations. I had been able to verbalise certain themes during the verbal check-in but the felt sensation in movement provided me with some more insight".

Learning more about the physical and emotional states of other group members captured a better picture of the climate of the group and situating oneself within the group received a lot of appraisals too, illustrated by participants' comments, such as: "Not everybody shares verbally. The movement has allowed me to understand the climate of the whole group", and "It's new for me and contradictory but it allows me to see more of the group and its climate". Members of the Focus Group added: "I don't think I have perceived the group as a space with different individuals, but rather I looked at the landscape or mood of the group as a whole", and "I have experienced some complete surprises".

Scores were slightly lower concerning the utility for connecting with others in the group: (36,4% complete agreement, 43,2% agreement, 13,6% neither agreeing or disagreeing, 4,6% disagreeing and 2,3% completely disagreeing).

One participant stated: "At one point there were only two of us in the same situation, all the other members represented different states. This seemed like an invitation for the two of us to get closer and move together".

The field notes of the researcher depict this event as follows:

> *I had suggested to choose closeness to the floor for those who were tired and higher levels for those who felt very awake. Participants vacillated between the two poles, moving up and down, extending certain parts of their body towards the ceiling, while others would fall towards the ground. A little group laid with their faces downwards on the floor, making the most of the contact with the ground underneath them. When I asked them to largen their general kinesphere and become aware of others in the group, smiles of sympathy and sighs were exchanged.*
>
> (*From* the field notes of the researcher)

One participant shared: "Being centred in my role in the group, my sensation is that it is not so easy to communicate and connect with others. But when you see where others are, you can connect empathically with those who are at the same level, or just in the opposite."

> *At the end of the first academic year students face the decision of either continuing with the entire master's training or continuing on with the postgraduate diploma, which is not a full training in DMT. Becoming a therapist or not may be a big decision for many, but also determining whether you continue the work with your group of peers or need to say good-bye. I suggested using one end of the studio for the masters' degree, and the other for the postgraduate degree and invited the students to place themselves between the two poles. Whereas certain students placed themselves clearly in one place, joining up with whom they found by their side while watching the rest of the group, others kept moving back and forth racing from one end to the other. At one stage somebody from the masters' end stretched out her hands and tried to keep back a peer who kept chasing about, and it seemed that with her intent to hug and hold back her friend she tried to show her affection and wish for the other to continue the training.*
>
> (*From* the field notes of the researcher)

A vivid discussion about how far the techniques could serve as a bridge between the verbal and nonverbal was sparked. Those who preferred sharing nonverbally mentioned, "I don't always like to share verbally", and "I am not sure how I could ever go back to verbal therapy after having discovered my connection with the movement". A member of the Focus Groups elaborated on this issue, saying

> "I find it stressful to listen to a verbal check-in with many participants feeling low. When peers share in movement it gives me a chance to see where they are at, but not having to take in all their problems."

However, the need for further explanation through verbalisation was mentioned, particularly with smaller and more advanced groups: "It has helped me to see the other person from a different place, promoting tolerance and respect, but requiring verbalisation in order to understand emotional states". A member of the Focus Group concluded: "Sometimes it has been rather stressful witnessing somebody in a particular state but not knowing why this person felt that way", and thus suggested altering verbal and nonverbal check-ins.

The second part of the questions connected more with issues of how to represent different physical and emotional states, touching on themes around movement observation and analysis.

The findings II: to what extent can different themes be represented through movement by an intercultural population?

The questions 11–30 of the questionnaire mainly dealt with the different proposals that had been suggested, for example, to represent happiness on a high level in space and sadness on a low level, anxiety with a lot of movement and physical well-being with open shapes, etc. The findings, thus, leave a trace of the lived experience of the 45 participants in terms of how to express certain inner states, given the variety of their personal body dimension and history, cultural, environment and geographical upbringing, as well as historic and socio-economic dimensions (Baruch et al, in revision). Participants were aged between 24 and 49 years and came from 14 different countries, including Catalonia and different parts of Spain, Portugal, Italy, Hungary, Poland, Greece, Israel, Chile, Ecuador, Mexico, Colombia, Argentina, Brazil and the USA.

Even though the responses from 45 participants do not allow for an accurate assessment in statistical terms, it still shows certain tendencies of how emotions are understood and expressed across cultures, extensively studied by movement therapists (for example Bartenieff & Lewis 1980; Chang 2006, 2009; De Tord & Bräuninger 2015; Kestenberg et al. 1999; Laban 1987; Panhofer et al. 2016) and neurolinguists (for example, Gibbs et al. 2004; Kövecses 2003; Lakoff 1987; Lakoff & Turner 1989).

Representing happiness on high levels in the space seemed to receive high accordance, just as is anchored in many languages, happy is up, like jumping for joy, feeling high, feeling in heaven or floating in the air. Upper levels in space were also associated with feeling awake or full of energy, linguistically connected to expressions like feeling lifted up, above the average or boosted up. On the contrary, low levels in the space were associated strongly with tired or sadness, confirming neurolinguistic concepts of a certain universality of the human body (Kövecses 2003). A great variety of human bodies seem to react to certain emotions with similar physical reactions, for example, to anger with a higher blood pressure, an accelerated heartbeat and a tenser muscle tone, or to sadness with a concave body torso, a lower glance and hanging shoulders. These concepts are anchored in our language with expressions such as feeling down, plunging deep, being on a low, downhearted, declining or dumping.

This rather universalist view of human bodies brings to mind Olivierto Toscani's controversial 1996 Benetton publicity, showing three hearts with the description white – black – yellow. It incentivises that no matter what colour we are, our most essential physicality is very similar. Albeit this historically essential contribution of outlining humankind's common features, DMT does not primarily deal with humans as *Körper* (corpus in Latin, the biological, the corpse), as one would expect from a physiotherapist or surgeon. More so, it addresses the lived body, in German the *Leib*, valuing its personal history and experience as an individual. Interestingly enough, the numbers of the survey support this deviation from a collective, unanimous explanation of movement. For example, the "happy is up" interpretation meets 7% disagreement and 5% neutral response, signalling the diversity of the group.

Theories of movement observation and analysis have been progressing from the universality to the particularity of movement meaning. Birdwhistle (1970) already pointed out the importance of context and social meaning of movement, distinguishing thus the isolated kinesic behaviour from its inevitable environment and underlying relationships. The survey has most certainly left a trace of this struggle: A large majority of the participants agreed with Bartenieff & Lewis' (1980) affirmation that a large personal kinesphere may be related to feeling secure, at ease or in control, embodying happiness and physical well-being through open body shapes. However, 5% disagreed and 9% neither agreed nor disagreed. Happiness is a very ambiguous word for me", one participant shared, probably hinting at the difficulty connecting with and sharing this feeling in the context of a university environment, in front of a lecturer within a particular group, etc. Many participants associated closed body shapes to insecurity, as described with the pin-like body shape (Bartenieff & Lewis 1980; Laban 1987). Thirty-one percent completely agreed and 43% agreed to associate closed body shapes to physical suffering (similar to the twisting shape) or unhappiness; however, 19% were neutral and 7% disagreed. One participant pointed out the particularity of the moment, saying, "Today, I did not perceive it that way".

How to express anxiety met even more varied responses. A lot of agitation and movement seemed to be quite appropriate for only half of the participants, whereas the other half did not seem to know or could not agree. "I perceive anxiety with a lot of movement, for me it's not about sitting still and nibbling my nails", a member of the Focus Group described. Lesser agreement was also found when associating higher levels in space to more mental states and lower levels in space to more physical states. One member of the Focus Groups reflected that she had enjoyed representing more physical states on a low level and more mental states on a high level, commenting, "I like the floor and have enjoyed becoming aware of this interpretation".

This brief exploration in the field of movement observation and analysis, thus, confirms that DMT moves beyond a universalist understanding of humans but rather adapts a socially and culturally inclusive way of working, considering differences such as race, ethnicity, class, ability, age, gender and sexual identity (Caldwell 2013). For the movement check-ins, it seems to be important to use simple binaries as a starting point from which to explore the particularities and uniqueness of each group and to plunge into the richness of its vocabulary as the group progresses. "Embodying different themes through movement" conceptualises the categories and exact numbers (Figure 2.1).

Discussing the findings with the focus group

The findings of the online survey were contrasted by an online Focus Group, consisting of six students who gathered for an hour to look at inherent group dynamics of the activity and reflect on further recommendations for the movement check-ins. It became evident that seeing others and being seen seemed an important theme. "I enjoyed being seen, not just feeling happy but also being able to share my happiness" is how one member of the group shared her need to be witnessed while expressing herself. Another member shared, "I felt more integrated in the group when I perceived others on the same level". However, sometimes participants felt awkward when representing certain states next to somebody in a very different mood, illustrated by the participant who said, "It was hard for me to embody happiness having somebody sad just next to me, it felt strange".

The fact of influencing each other was brought up as well, for example, one member of the focus group commented, "Sometimes I found it hard as I felt that my body wanted to be in two poles at the same time. I felt empathy with different people I watched, and torn apart between distinct shades". The idea of undertaking the activity with closed eyes, in order to get in touch

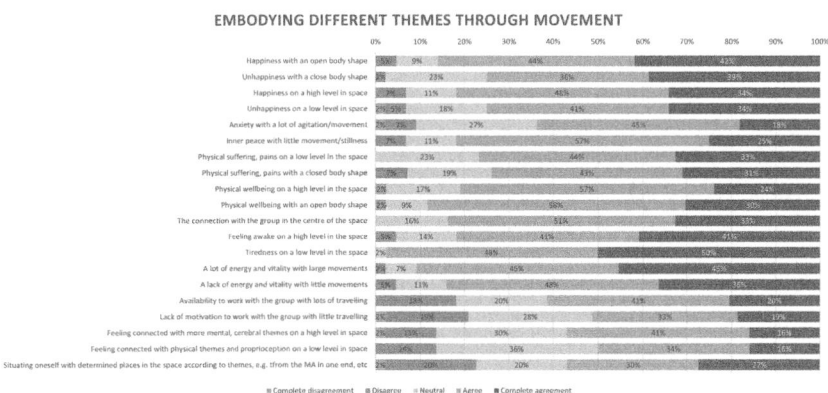

Figure 2.1 Embodying different themes through movement.

with one's inner states, emerged, similar to Authentic Movement, an im-provisational movement practice that works with free association and closed eyes. The phantasy of not being influenced by others seemed tempting, but members soon agreed that the outcome would be certainly affected by group dynamics and the fact of being witnessed, just like in Authentic Movement (Payne 2017).

Another main subject that emerged through the Focus Group was the possibility of not sharing anything at all, for example, one participant said, "There is no possibility of not sharing, only being physically present is a state-ment". Others pointed out that even in verbal groups, silent members em-bodied their states of being through their physical presence and their silence. It was, thus, proposed to allow for a neutral position that expressed the need of not wishing to share, as one participant articulated, "For me, allowing for a neutral point is very important".

The limitations of the activity were also discussed, and a mixture of movement and verbal check-ins were recommended for smaller groups, the members of which had actually more intimacy and lesser need for such a directive activity. Limitations for certain populations were considered, for example, for those who suffer from a severe body-mind split, profound disability or autism. However, participants of the Focus Group had ap-plied the movement check-in with mental health patients and clients with learning disabilities, where the clear suggestions and timing of the activity had worked really well. It was further suggested to integrate objects that could help to sign certain body parts that may be aching or aid all sorts of expression. However, all participants agreed that they saw no use in learning a kind of nonverbal code prior to being able to participate in the activity, as this is sometimes proposed for patients who might not respond to traditional methods. More so, emerging group dynamics should be ob-served cautiously, in order to develop a group's own culture and language and learn how to move beyond binaries.

Conclusions

This chapter has aimed at presenting and revising the technique of checking in using bodily movement. Inspired by the Post-Cartesian notion to unite bodies and minds, the verbal and the nonverbal, this approach had been de-veloped at the Autonomous University of Barcelona for medium- and large-sized groups. Forty-five students from two different promotions and a small follow-up Focus Group evaluated and shared their experience of the move-ment check-ins. At first sight, the numbers of the Survey Monkey Question-naire seemed too generic, unanimously praising the exit of the technique, and thus a bit one dimensional. The field notes of the researcher, the com-ments and discussion with the students helped to bring the numbers alive, drawing attention to additional vital aspects of the technique, and furthering its educational and therapeutic implications.

The movement check-ins were shown to be useful, particularly in order to pay attention to one's own physical and emotional conditions, to learn about the group's different states and recognise common themes. However, processing these would require more time, experience and trust. The suggestions of how to embody certain themes in movement have been appreciated as rather useful, such as locating happiness up and sadness down, connecting open body shapes with physical well-being and closed body shapes with physical suffering, shyness or ill-being (Barteniefff & Lewis 1980; Laban 1987). However, both the numbers and the feedback clearly showed that the proposals need to develop from a binary orientation to a broader spectrum, integrating the particularity of the experience and valuing the individual beyond a generic, universalist view. Body language is tightly linked to one's personal history and body dimension; one's cultural, environmental and geographical upbringing, as well as historic and socio-economic dimensions (Baruch et al. in revision, Chang 2006, 2009). It needs to be considered within its context, albeit an academic setting, a therapy or peer group. Furthermore, it seemed important to mix verbal and nonverbal check-ins to attend a maximum of needs and variety: allowing for movement where words have fallen short and allowing for verbalisation where movement cannot be clear enough.

As Shalem-Zafari & Grosu (2016) confirm:

> (...) DMT integrates insights from nonverbal experience, from verbal discussion, and from cognitive observation analysis. These all have their place in comprising this complex profession and contribute to a certain balance within the practice of DMT. This balance allows both for deep self-expression, rooted in the body and movement, and for the ability to understand this expression.
>
> (670)

Future research could aim at evaluating the technique with larger numbers of participants or applying it with different client groups such as learning disabilities, third age, mental health patients, children, or all kinds of populations where wording one's emotional and bodily experience seems to be challenging. It is hoped that the technique stimulates all kinds of psychotherapists to observe and enhance their client's movement expressions and integrate their nonverbal language, whenever words fall short.

Note

1 The middle-sized or median group (de Maré et al. 1991) with about 20–40 members bridges the small family-sized, tribal group with the large hunter-type or society-like group (Schulamit 2017). At the DMT training in Barcelona, groups may vary from 7 to 60 members, depending on the subject and methodology.

References

Bartenieff, I. & Lewis, D. (1980). *Body movement – coping with the environment*. New York, Gordon and Breach.

Baruch, Y., Kazamiaki, E., Kokontini, M. & Panhofer, H. (2021). When cultures move: a comparison between two cultural groups (Greece and Israel) based on a Movement Profile Analysis. Thesis in partial fulfilment of the Master's Programme in Dance Movement Therapy at the Autonomous University in Barcelona.

Bergold, J. & Thomas, St. (2012). Participatory research methods: a methodological approach in motion. *Historical Social Research / Historische Sozialforschung*, 37 (4), pp. 191–222.

Birdwhistle, R. (1970). *Kinesics and context: essays on body motion communication*. Philadelphia, University of Pennsylvania Press.

Caldwell, C. (2013). Diversity issues in movement observation and assessment. *American Journal of Dance Therapy*, 35 (2), pp. 183–200.

Chang, M. (2006). How do dance/movement therapists bring awareness of race, ethnicity, and cultural diversity into their practice? In S.C. Koch & I. Bräuninger (eds.), *Advances in dance/movement therapy. Theoretical perspectives and empirical findings*. Berlin, Logos, pp. 192–205.

Chang, M. (2009). Cultural consciousness and the global context of dance/movement therapy. In S. Chaiklin & H. Wengrower (eds.), *The art and science of dance/movement therapy: life is dance*. New York, Routledge, pp. 299–312.

Curtis, S. (2002). Providing dance movement therapy within a mainstream school. In Bannister, A. & Huntington, A. (eds.), Communicating with children and adolescents: Action for change. London, Jessica Kingsley, pp. 114–127.

de Maré, P., Piper, R. & Thompson, S. (1991). *Koinonia: from hate, through dialogue to culture in the large group*. London: Karnac Books.

Denham, M.A. & Onwuegbuzie, A.J. (2013). Beyond words: using nonverbal communication data in research to enhance thick description and interpretation. *International Journal of Qualitative Methods*, 12, pp. 670–696.

De Tord, P.D., & Bräuninger, I. (2015). Grounding: theoretical application and practice in dance movement therapy. *The Arts in Psychotherapy*, 43, pp. 16–22.

Dietrich-Hartwell, R., Goodhill, S. & Koch, S. (2020). Dance/movement therapy with resettled refugees: a guideline and framework based on empirical data. *The Arts in Psychotherapy*, 69, p. 101664.

Gibbs, R.W., Lenz, P.C.L. & Francozo, E. (2004). Metaphor is grounded in embodied experience. *Journal of Pragmatics*, 36, pp. 1189–1210.

Kestenberg, A., Loman, S., Lewis P. & Sossin, K.M. (1999). *The meaning of movement developmental and clinical perspectives of the Kestenberg movement profile*. Amsterdam, Gordon and Breach Publishers, 2nd edition Routledge.

Kitzinger, J. (1995). Education and debate. Qualitative research: introducing focus groups. *British Medical Journal*, 311, pp. 299–302.

Kövecses, Z. (2003). *Metaphor and emotion. Language, culture, and body in human feeling*. Cambridge, Cambridge University Press.

Laban, R. (1987). *El Dominio del Movimiento*. Madrid, Ed. Fundamentos.

Lakoff, G. (1987). Image metaphors. *Metaphor and Symbol*, 2 (3), pp. 219–222.

Lakoff, G. & Turner, M. (1989). *More than cool reason: a field guide to poetic metaphor*. Chicago, The University of Chicago Press.

Meekums, B. (2002). *Dance movement therapy: creative therapies in practice.* London: Sage.

Meekums, B. (2008). Developing emotional literacy through individual dance movement therapy: a pilot study. *Emotional and Behavioural Difficulties,* 13 (2), pp. 1741–2692.

Moore, C.L. & Yamamoto, K. (2011, 2nd edition). *Beyond words. Movement observation and analysis.* London, Gordon and Breach.

Panhofer, H. & Rodríguez Cigaran, S. (2005). La danza movimiento terapia: una nueva profesión se introduce en España. In H. Panhofer (ed.), *El cuerpo en psicoterapia.* Barcelona: Gedisa, pp. 49–95.

Panhofer, H. (2011). Langugaged and non-languaged ways of knowing in counselling and psychotherapy. *British Journal of Guidance and Counselling,* 39 (5), pp. 455–470.

Panhofer, H., García, M.E. & Zelaskowski, P. (2014). The challenge of working with embodied, emotional consciousness in the context of a university-based dance movement therapy training. *The Arts in Psychotherapy,* 41, pp. 115–119.

Panhofer, H., Bräuninger, I. & Zelaskowski, P. (2016). Dance movement therapy training: the challenges of interculturality and cross-cultural communication within a diverse student group-analytic large group. In D. Dokter & M. Hills De Zárate (eds.), *Intercultural arts therapies research. Issues and methodologies.* London, Routledge, pp. 56–74.

Payne, H. (2017). The psycho-neurology of embodiment with examples from authentic movement and Laban Movement Analysis. *The American Journal for Dance Therapy,* 39, pp. 163–178.

Savidaki, M., Demirtoka, S. & Rodríguez-Jiménez (2020). Re-inhabiting one's body: A pilot study on the effects of dance movement therapy on body image and alexithymia in eating disorders. *Journal of Eating Disorders,* 8 (22), https://doi.org/10.1186/s40337-020-00296-2.

Schulamit, G. (2017). The Median Group. GAD Blog. https://groupanalyticsociety.co.uk/the-median-group/.

Shalem-Zafari & Grosu, E.F. (2016). DMT, past and present: how history can inform current supervision. *The European Proceedings of Social & Behavioural Sciences EpSBS.* http://dx.doi.org/10.15405/epsbs.2016.12.81.

Valdivia, M.E. (2010). A psychoanalytic perspective of endings in therapy: a Dance Movement Psychotherapy case study. *Body, Movement and Dance in Psychotherapy,* 5 (1), pp. 75–87.

3 Arts-based research and self-reflexive autobiographical performance

Ditty Dokter

Mijn landen komen samen weer
verdronken over Doggerland
geen grenzen verdelen meer
moet ik dat echt wensen heer?

(from Fluid Borders: own lyrics to Boudewijn de Groot Waterdrager (1968))
   English translation:

My countries may soon join again
drowned over Doggerland
no more borders between them
should I really wish for that?

Introduction

This chapter outlines the autobiographical performance concept and the arts-based research methodology used to inquire about its impact. It describes a triptych of autobiographical performances devised improvisationally via Amerta movement improvisation (Bloom et al. 2014). As an older migrant the inquiry was an embodied expression of 'narratives of home' by a transnational (Walsh & Nare 2016). The findings of the arts-based study will be contextualised in literature and a previous phenomenological inquiry about self-reflexive performance in arts therapies training (Dokter & Gersie 2016).

As a drama and dance movement therapist, my practice is psychodynamic (Karkou & Sanderson 2006). As a migrant I bridge countries, as an arts psychotherapist I bridge modalities; this brings challenges and rewards. Embodiment as a catalyst for change provides the connection (Dokter 2016).

Self-reflexive performance is defined as a self-referential personal performance where the content consists of material from the lives of the performers (Pendzik et al. 2016). Rycroft (1983) queried almost 40 years ago whether its purpose was merely the 'advertising of a longstanding ego' (193) and emphasised the need for a reflexive practice that aimed at self-discovery. The intersection between self-referential performance as an art form and a therapeutic

DOI: 10.4324/9781003222484-3

method is a place of meeting and departure. The potentially healing aspects of autobiographical performance may be associated with the feminist and political inception of the genre, aiming to fuel the performer's sense of agency, underlining transformative possibilities and offering a stage to public presentations of the personal (Pendzik 2016). There are connections to autoethnographic performance, which is also socio-political-gender oriented and tends to have a 'social awareness agenda' (Saldana 2011: 13). Autobiographical performance as self-referential performance can connect with personal healing and refers to artists' work dealing with traumatic life events as 'acts of recovery' (Heddon 2008: 54).

Methodology

Other research into self-reflexive performance I took part in was phenomenological (Dokter & Gersie 2016; Jacques 2019). This researched other people's experiences. To research my own experience of self-reflexive performance, I chose arts-based research to privilege the movement exploration as data collection and performance as presentation of findings.

'The definitive aspects of artistic methods of research in the arts therapies are art-making as data gathering, data analysis and as presentation of findings' (Hervey 2000: 45). Crucial to my research was embodied artistic inquiry, a methodology that may use art / dance making to collect data, analyse data and present findings; which acknowledges a creative research process; is shaped by the aesthetic values of the researcher and may draw upon embodied experiences of the researcher and participants as sources of information and understanding (Hervey 2012).

In this type of practice-led arts-based research, data took the form of words (research notes / journals) and arts products (in my case tapestry weavings, drawings and crystallisations) (Miller 2014). The journaling and drawings focus on the embodiment experience. Woven tapestries are a parallel practice exploring landscape qualities of both 'home' countries (www.whitwellweaving.co.uk).

My data collection involved working as a member of a creative project group for a year for each of the performances: improvising through movement, journaling the movement explorations and devising a performance as a culmination of those explorations. The vignettes used in the presentation of findings come from the journaling notes (Dokter 2021). The findings were disseminated in three performances entitled Finding Home (2015), Come or Go (2017) and Fluid borders (2021). The first part of the triptych 'Finding home' focused on migration and mortality. I have written elsewhere about the illness recovery aspect of that work (Dokter 2021; Dokter et al. 2020). 'Come or Go' focused on the impact of the Brexit referendum on an EU migrant, whilst 'Fluid borders' explored the experience of migrant mother-daughter intergenerational links impacted by pandemic and citizenship issues. The themes from the movement-based explorations were illness, mortality and accepting limitations; migration and borders; home and belonging.

These themes emerged in the embodied inquiry as radical adult transitions (Hervey 2012). A radical adult transition is a major change made after a period of stability in an adult's life that affects relationships, identity and life direction. The movement form for the embodied inquiry was Amerta movement (Bloom et al. 2014; Reeve 2021), which is distinct from other movements and somatic practices in that it asks the practitioner to follow their own experiences, especially the sensory-motoric. Practitioners interact with both environment and self, whilst being in communication with the cultural heritage and personalities of fellow movers. A relationship with the past comes alive as part of the present. The practice has roots in Vipassana (mindfulness), daily life movement, non-stylised movement and a Javanese meditation form called Sumarah.

Arts–based research project

In an embodied pilot post-cancer diagnosis and treatment, I needed to explore the changes in my movement profile. I am now registered disabled, the treatment affected my joints and mobility. The following vignette from my journal illustrates the transition to recover agency in my movement.

Two of us move together in a sea cave, we alternate moving. I tap with my stick against the cave ceiling and the boulders around me: Can I move, can I climb or am I stuck here, can I get out? Slowly, at times crawling, at times using my sticks, I manage to traverse the obstacles to the big flat boulder at the entrance of the cave. I heave myself up it to standing. I can stand without my sticks facing the sea (Figure 3.1).

I embarked on the first part of my inquiry with the following research question: Can embodied inquiry aid a process of radical transition as recovery? A secondary question was about changes to migrant identity in the face of mortality and life-threatening illness: What is the place where I can live (dis) abled and have a home to die? The illness experience raised new questions about belonging. The autobiographical work related to personal healing and dealing with traumatic events as an 'act of recovery' (Heddon 2008: 54), but it also had wider social echoes. Migrants drowning whilst traversing the sea recalled my professional experience of working with refugees (Dokter 1998, 2000), connecting the personal, professional and political. The inquiry culminated in a performance with an invited audience, in a wild garden on top of a cliff facing the sea. As props I had asked the group that I worked with to contribute birds' nests vacated by their owners. After embodying my own migration journey from young adult to older adulthood I ask them to find a place for their nest in the garden and weave a three-dimensional web between them. I accompany the movement by singing Mijn vlakke land / My flat country (Brel 1962) in contrast to the landscape around me to emphasise the contrasts. I sing in my first language to enable the non-Dutch speaking audience members to experience the sense of linguistic and landscape alienation (English translation in the programme). The performance concludes with a chant evoking the call of a spiritual home.

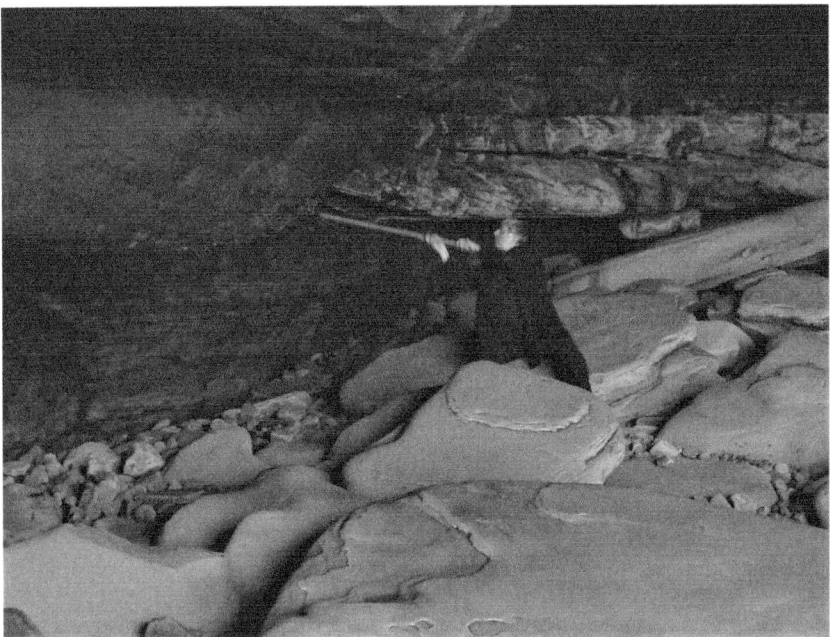

Figure 3.1 Photograph of Ditty Dokter's performance.

Change of language and landscape, together with the question of welcome in the adopted country, as well as the ability to continue / find a way of expressing spirituality / religion are all aspects of identity impacted by the experience of migration. I was interested to note that the radical transition of illness and disability required revisiting previous radical transitions such as migration.

The second period of inquiry took place during the Brexit referendum year. The inquiry shifted from a more personal act of recovery to a more explicit connection that the personal is political. 'Come or Go' continued the theme of radical transition as there would be a period of choice whether to stay or go. The referendum started a period of limbo for EU citizens in the UK (Remigi et al. 2017). There was some agency in the choice of residence for me, unlike refugees whose period of limbo waiting for refugee status can be one of profound hopelessness (Callaghan 1998). The referendum split the UK into those who voted to remain against those voting to leave, with a 48% minority on the leave side. To restore my sense of agency, I wanted to share the impact of this hostile environment to immigration on my own sense of belonging. Could I ever be other than out of place (Said 2000)? Could I find a way to resist the power of a hostile host (Fang 2020)?

A vignette from a group movement improvisation embodies my felt experience:

> I move along the edge of the group, trying to connect from the outside – watching with a sense of 'outsiderness'. I do not feel I can engage in the group play although I can make connections with individuals, but after each individual movement connection I say goodbye – move on.

This inquiry aimed explicitly to create a public performance in an area with a strong 'leave' vote. I named it 'Come or Go'. Instead of using existing nests provided by others as in 'Finding home', I wove a willow boat and the beach was the public performance site location. The flux between land and sea, the constantly shifting landscape reflected my questions about belonging and welcome. Although my mobility had improved, the surface of pebbles made walking hazardous and I needed helpers to facilitate my entry in and exit from the sea. This reflected my own ambivalence whether I had steady ground under my feet in the face of Brexit, was I assisted to leave or to remain? The timing of the promenade performance was at the change of the tide where the sea starts to return and the land disappears.

It is a very blustery September day when I meet with my audience on Charmouth beach. Using my sticks, I draw COME on one and Go on the other side of the outlet pipe on the beach. I am aware that my 'known' audience has gathered underneath the quay, whilst strangers witness me from above or walk past me, mostly giving me a wide birth. I walk with my sticks over the outlet pipe towards the lower audience group and invite them to join me to walk the words as a path, first Come then Go. My woven boat awaits at Go and I say goodbye to the group by giving a sprig of flowers to each person in the circle. I pick up the boat, lift it on my shoulder and walk across the beach to where the river flows across it to the sea. The audience has walked with me and I apologetically explain that I know the boat is probably not seaworthy but that 'if you have to go, you have to go'. The audience moves me by spontaneously weaving the flowers I gave them into the willow boat. My helper supports me in trying to launch the boat, then in the sea itself. At the edge of the beach, I leave my stick and I swim out alone with the boat. It proves not seaworthy in the waves and capsizes, despite my best efforts to keep it (and me) afloat. Floating on its side the boat returns, as do I (Figure 3.2).

I sing 'Ik zou wel eens willen weten/ I really would like to know' (de Corte 1955) each verse in Dutch and English at different places during the promenade (at Come by the sea, at the launch of the boat in the river and on my final return to the beach). The final verse identifies with the corroding cliffs at Charmouth, not knowing how long they will live and belong or when they will disappear.

The performance took place a month after a small company of migrant students and staff performed their autobiographical experiences as Nomadians theatre company with the production 'Welcome question mark' at the Edinburgh fringe (Carr et al. 2017), one of many performances around the theme of Brexit that summer. The audience response was mostly receptive. The solo performance on a windswept and wet public beach in Dorset felt

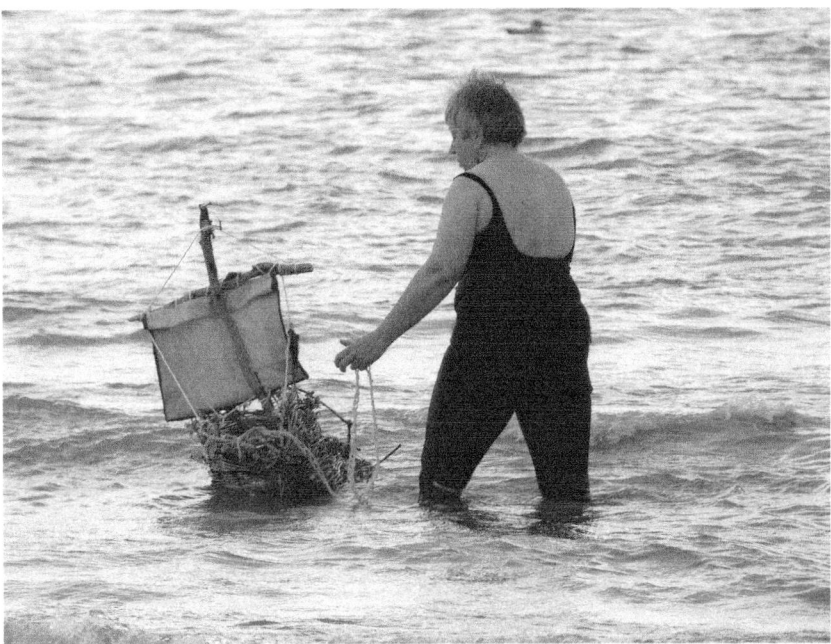

Figure 3.2 Photograph of Ditty Dokter's performance.

more akin to the hostile migration environment created by the UK government (Fang 2020).

The third and final component of the arts-based inquiry completed the series. The performance was titled Fluid borders and was devised whilst applying for dual citizenship during a pandemic lockdown. The lockdown started during a period of bereavement for my mother, who died February 2020, whilst my daughter had moved across to the Netherlands in September 2019. Its initial theme was around staying/having to stay and was devised in the context of the impact of the pandemic on migrants, the implementation of Brexit and applying for settled status and citizenship. Themes emerged around fluid and rigid borders in relation to migrant identity. The site-specific performance took place eight months after the implementation of Britain leaving the EU, five years after the Brexit referendum, having completed the citizenship process. Dutch law changed recently to enable dual citizenship. My sense of belonging is – with ambivalences – in both countries. Not being able to travel back and forwards between my two countries during the pandemic reminded me yet again of the experience of my refugee clients for whom this was not an option either, which often exacerbated their sense of alienation and loss. Lockdown, Brexit, the loss of my mother and (temporary) loss of my daughter created yet another period of radical transition.

As the first period of this final inquiry occurred during lockdown and the group met on zoom, I decided to make a film. This connected my mother as a skater and myself as a swimmer through the objects of my mother's old Dutch wooden skates and my swimming in a local river from a place called Skaters' meadow; it connected my two homes of east Anglia and the eastern Netherlands.

I struggle with my feeling of 'having to stay' and ask fellow group members to embody staying by moving on the spot and by moving in a small delineated space. I witness their movements on screen and they share their drawings / writings about the experience with me. One group member shares how she discovered a new spot in a very familiar space, excitedly writing, 'there is scope for composition in the tiniest space!', whilst another (a fellow migrant) shares her entry into staying as 'going in and out again', but then also 'it is surprising how much you can do in one spot'. This contrasts with my own experience of wanting to challenge the boundaries when the space I enter is smaller than expected, but also a realisation that when entering a space I tend to look far, whilst when I look near, something changes and I can find space.

In the performance, I contrast the skating and swimming in the film with a live embodiment of my feet moving frustratedly on a small rug, another object that used to belong to my mother. I sing live whilst the film shows my hands in breast stroke through the river. I welcome the audience by showing them the river systems and North sea connecting my two homes via a nautical chart wrapped around my body.

During the arts-based inquiry with the project group members, we explored embodiment in small spaces, screen focus on individual body parts such as feet and hands. We found that sharing and moving with objects in the space was a way of sharing the space we were moving in. I asked group members to move some of my themes to be able to reflect on my own experience and bridge the sense of isolation with each of us in our zoom boxes. The narrower focus in a locality was facilitated by lockdown. Sharing these with each other, one project member said to me – in an attempt to comfort my sense of distance – 'but you swim in the rivers that connect you, so you are not really cut off'. This comment became the leitmotif for my final inquiry. The text after the abstract shows some of the new lyrics about fluid borders to the water carrier song (de Groot 1968).

The binary nature of Come or Go became integrated in an embodiment of fluid borders.

In the performance itself, some of the realities of rigid borders were re-enacted by crossing from the safe haven of a village hall across several thresholds. One of these included being asked for papers and being divided into one group or another according to the colour of your paper. The group was guided to different sides of the river, where I embodied the sense of travelling back and forwards in movement and by weaving a web across the stream. The audience became my important others on both sides of the water.

The intergenerational connections from mother to daughter / daughter to mother eased my sense of loss, whilst the transformation of a hostile environment to a connecting network of relationships facilitated transformation of alienation and agency in making choices. Radical transitions of death and migration could be shared and transformed from a sense of passivity / oppression to active giving and receiving.

Oppressive nationalist systems and hostile environments do not change, but at the beginning of this tryptich inquiry I started from a position of anger at oppression and a sense of helplessness / having been 'done to' (in both cancer and migrant treatment). My anger at the systemic institutional nature of oppression has not changed; I choose to engage with various forms of activism. On a more personal level, I am starting to accept a sense of transnational belonging and gratitude for the possibility of transformation. Illness and mortality (my own and that of my parents), as well as migration (my own and my daughter's) have been radical transitions.

Placing the findings of my arts-based inquiry into a wider context, I will now discuss literature in relation to the themes and other research into autobiographical performance.

Migration and identity; performance content and forms

Content: themes and their link to literature (see endnote 2)

The right to freedom of movement was established in the 1948 Declaration of Universal Human Rights, Article 13 (United Nations 1948) which meant the right to move and stay within the borders of each state, as well as the right to leave and return to the country. Paradoxically, the history of migration, which is a long one, is a history of controls on the movement of all but a wealthy elite (Trilling 2018). Many countries have long histories of migration, be it out or in. Both my countries, Britain and the Netherlands, have a long history of immigration (Winder 2004), as well as emigration beyond the history of colonialisation, which of course is part of this (Wekker 2016).

International migration has had a significant impact on the formulation and content of foreign policy. The framing of European integration has parallelled xenophobia, prejudice and right-wing populism (Kende & Kreko 2020). Insecurities about being able / having a right to stay can create discrimination and exploitation, whilst dual citizens / multinationals are viewed with suspicion and in certain circumstances can have their citizenship revoked (Cowan 2021; Trilling 2018). Migration takes effort, for many migrants the poor social conditions and loss of status / cultural identity takes a toll on their psychological health. I wrote 20 years ago 'It is not simply a matter of geographical and cultural dislocation, the adjustment and inevitable stresses of migration' (Dokter 1998: 146). An important issue is the ongoing response of and to the white host society, its values and institutions. The ongoing response of the white host society seems to have become ever more hostile, denying the benefits migrants bring to both their host and birth countries.

A transnational is between cultures, situated within the cross-cultural encounter rather than dwelling above it. Said speaks to the merits of positioning ourselves on the margins 'I actually prefer not being quite right and being out of place' (Said 2000: 295). The discourse of the in-between cultural subject can be silent on how unequal power relations impact the experience of in-betweenness. Belonging and attachment are complex for intercultural / transnational subjects. There is an assumption that you do not belong if you are black in a white context, as a migrant there can be an issue of being able to 'pass' on skin colour. Invisibility can be a form of assimilation, denying difference, a pressure to 'integrate'. Belonging is as much in the individual as it is within the communal context. Blackwell (2005) in his work with refugees discusses the importance of addressing the political, cultural, interpersonal and intrapsychic level of both the client and the therapist's experience in therapy. His understanding of working with the unconscious in therapy provides an interesting perspective on same and other: 'If we take seriously our professed belief in the unconscious…, we are always, in some important sense "other" to ourselves. Thus, whenever we talk about "us" and "them" we are always more "other" to each other than we like to imagine, and "they" are always another collection of others, not only more "other" to each other, but also more like ourselves than we are prepared to concede' (2005: 17).[1]

Research into the psychosocial effects and stresses on immigrants and minority groups highlight both the psychological opportunities (Beltsiou 2016) and the risks of alienation (Dokter 1998, 2008). This is true for both therapists and clients. The response of the surrounding community to these opportunities and stresses effects the sense of (not) belonging, especially if that response is one of inequity and exclusion. Social, political, cultural and historical contexts shape the psychological experience of migration and with it the encounter and interaction between clients and therapists and the possibility of intergenerational trauma being re-enacted between the therapist and client (Layton 2017).

Form in self-reflexive autobiographical performance

As a dramatherapy and dance therapy trainer, I was interested to note that there were similarities in the way I gave form to what trainees said about their autobiography experiences. In parallel to the arts-based work, I co-researched – through phenomenological interviewing – the impact of self-reflexive autobiographical performance during dramatherapy training (Dokter & Gersie 2016). Graduates from three training programmes, ranging from newly qualified to those qualifying 25 years ago, were asked to reflect on the impact of that performance on their identity as an arts therapist. All participants identified diversity-related issues as important to their explorations (disability, ethnicity, nationality, class, age, religion, sexual orientation). They articulated a sense of agency in being able to share their differences and having them witnessed by others. As researchers, we asked about the form participants chose to share their personal material; whether they chose metaphorical or direct representation and what the impact was of a known or unknown audience. Pendzik identifies the oppression / liberation paradigm in autobiographical performance and studies the stage metaphors of the body-as-evidence and body-of-evidence: 'The dialogue between form and context is always dialectical' (Pendzik 2016: 59).

In my arts-based findings about mortality and the ageing body, the search for a form that could communicate / share these experiences in a way that conveyed agency meant accepting aids: material, human and environmental to help connect form and content. Many audience members commented on the impact of climate change refugees; conflicts and migration became a wider political context. My relationship with the audience was ambivalent: were they the oppressive other or helpers? Could I accept as allies those whom I perceived as potentially hostile? I was interested that throughout the three performances audience participation evolved from embodying fellow exiles, to embodying both allies and Brexiteers, to embodying separated important others. The relationship between mover and witness is part of the transformational process when inquiring about the body as a catalyst for change. The interaction with fellow inquirer movers throughout strengthened a sense of agency and being able to make choices, as well as a sense of common humanity.

Conclusion

In arts-based research, the concept of translation is a possible evaluation criterion; it means the transformation of one form of knowledge into another. How does the language of art affect the idea? I have aimed to be explicit about the research process (another criterion). Trustworthiness and authenticity meant staying close to personal lived experience, whilst audience response was a final important marker for the impact of the performances (Leavy 2020).

Inquiring with others and being witnessed by others about the themes of isolation and alienation held seeds for transformation. The role of movement and embodiment when re-finding agency in an ageing 'dis' abled body can be equally transformative. Finding creativity when the experience is one of destructiveness is crucial for the body to become a catalyst for change.

Acknowledgements

I want to profoundly thank Sandra Reeve and the members of the Amerta project groups who supported this work, as well as my students and colleagues at Anglia Ruskin University, especially Mandy Carr; David Tatem, as always, for his unstinting support in ever so many ways.

Note

1 Further information can be found in Dokter, D. and Sajnani, N. (2022). *Intercultural dramatherapy. Imaginings across intersectional differences.* London, Routledge. In press.

References

Beltsiou, J. (ed) (2016). *Immigration in psychoanalysis. Locating ourselves.* London: Routledge.

Blackwell, D. (2005). *Counselling and psychotherapy with refugees.* London: Jessica Kingsley.

Bloom, K., Galanter, M. & Reeve, S. (eds) (2014). *Embodied lives. Reflections in the influence of Suprapto Suryodarma and Amerta movement.* Axminster: Triarchy Press.

Brel, J. (1962). Mijn vlakke land. https:m.youtube.com/watch?v=DEIDVP1PUBw.

Callaghan, K. (1998). In limbo. In Dokter, D. (ed) *Arts therapists, refugees and migrants* (pp. 25–40). London: Jessica Kingsley.

Carr M., Dokter, D., Martin, J., Mullen-Williams, J., Nemeckova, S. & Yeni, N. (2017). Welcome question mark. Performances 10–17 August, Edinburgh Fringe festival, Edinburgh. Cowan, L. (2021). Border nation. A story of migration. London: Pluto Press.

de Corte, J. (1957). Ik zou wel eens willen weten. https:m.youtube.com/watch?v=cFIJ6EvicFO.

de Groot, B. (1968). De waterdrager. https:m.youtube.com?watch?v=ISGUKBXq-So.

Dokter, D. (ed) (1998). *Arts therapists refugees and migrants. Reaching across borders.* London: Jessica Kingsley.

Dokter, D. (2000/1). Intercultural dramatherapy practice: a research history. *Dramatherapy* 22(3), pp. 3–8.

Dokter, D. (2008). Immigrant mental health. Acculturation and the response of the UK 'host'. In Dent-Brown, K. & Finklestein, M. (eds) *Psychosocial stress in immigrants and in members of minority groups as a factor of terrorist behaviour* (pp. 168–178). Amsterdam: IOS Press.

Dokter, D. (2016). Embodiment. In Jennings, S. & Holmwood, C. (eds) *The international handbook of dramatherapy.* London: Routledge.

Dokter, D. (2021). The transformative body. In Reeve, S. (ed) *Body and awareness* (pp. 219–232). Axminster: Triarchy Press.

Dokter, D. & Gersie, A. (2016). A retrospective study of autobiographical performance during dramatherapy training. In Pendzik et al. op cit (pp. 181–198).

Dokter, D., Lea-Weston, L. & Thornewood, T. (2020). Secondary traumatisation and therapist illness. In A. Chesner & S. Lykou (eds) *Arts therapies and trauma* (pp. 143–154). London: Routledge.

Fang, N. (2020). Feeling/being out of place: psychic defence against the hostile environment. https://www.ed.ac.uk/health/research/centres/ccri/first-thursday-seminars-20-21/feeling-out-of-place Accessed 20.9.2021.

Heddon, D. (2008). *Autobiography and performance.* New York, Palgrave MacMillan.

Hervey, L.W. (2000). *Artistic inquiry in dance movement therapy: Creative alternatives for research.* Springfield Il: Charles C Thomas.

Hervey, L.W. (2012). Embodied artistic inquiry. In Cruz, R. & Berroll, C. (eds) *Dance movement therapists in action.* Springfield, IL, Charles C. Thomas 2nd ed.

Jacques, J. (2019). Investigation into the production of meaning in autobiographical performance in dramatherapy. *Arts in Psychotherapy* 69 (2020), p. 101659.

Karkou V. & Sanderson, P. (2006). *Arts therapies. A research based map of the field.* Amsterdam: Elsevier.

Kende, A. & Kreko, P. (2020). Xenophobia, prejudice, and right-wing populism in East-Central Europe. August 2020 *Current Opinion in Behavioral Sciences* 34, pp. 29–33. DOI:10.1016/j.cobeha.2019.11.011.

Layton, L. (2017). Racialised enactments and normative unconscious processes. Where haunted identities meet. In Grand, S. & Salberg, J. (eds) *Transgenerational trauma and the other. Dialogues across history and difference.* London: Routledge.

Leavy, P. (2020). Method meets art. Artsbased research in practice 3rd ed. New York: Guilford Press.

Miller, K. (2014). Amerta movement and archeology. In Bloom, K., Galanter, M. & Reeve, S. (eds) *Embodied lives. Reflections in the influence of Suprapto Suryodarma and Amerta movement.* Axminster: Triarchy Press.

Pendzik, S., Emunah, R. & Johnson, D.R. (eds) (2016). *The self in performance.* New York: Palgrave McMillan.

Reeve, S. (ed) (2021). *Body and awareness.* Axminster: Triarchy Press.

Remigi, E., Martin, V. & Sykes, T. (2017). In limbo. Brexit testimonies from EU citizens in the UK. www.OurBrexitBlog.eu.

Rycroft, C. (1983). *Psychoanalysis and beyond.* London: Hogarth Press.

Said, E. (2000). *Out of place.* New York: Vintage Books.

Saldana, J. (2011). *Ethnotheatre. Research from page to stage.* Walnut Creek, CA: Left Coast Press.

Trilling, D. (2018). *Lights in the distance. Exile and refuge at the borders of Europe.* London: Picador.

Walsh, K. & Nare, L. (eds) (2016). *Transnational migration and home in older age.* London: Routledge.

Wekker, G. (2016). *White innocence. Paradoxes of colonialism and race.* London: Duke University Press.

Winder, R. (2004). *Bloody foreigners. The story of immigration to Britain.* London: Little Brown.

4 Kinaesthetic entanglements and creative immersion in embodied performance

Marina Rova

An unexpected…performance

Recently, I escorted a family member to a general hospital for a lengthy medical examination. As I sat in the hospital waiting area, I became a witness to what became a rather distressing scene: A woman pushed the stroller of a screaming toddler up and down the long corridor again and again and again. The first time they walked past I was shaken out of my reverie, my thoughts paused mid-air (so to speak). I sat quietly listening as the toddler's cries disappeared into the distance. I let out a sigh and reached for a book in my bag. And then I heard the crying again, steadily growing in volume, as the pair made their way back, reaching its crescendo as they walked in front of me. This time, I was actively engaged in my witnessing as I watched them disappear round the corner. I noticed a wave of dread in my body. Is the baby in pain? Back they were a third time, the baby screaming louder, crying "mummy, mummy". The woman kept walking purposefully, eyes straight ahead. She was on a mission. I could not read her expression behind her mask. Is she in pain? Off they went again. I was now aware of my affective and somatic responses. I found myself checking the corridor in anticipation of their return and wondered whether I should move to another waiting area to allow them some privacy. Before I could make up my mind, they were back. I felt a piercing sensation in my stomach and I felt my eyes moisten. What was happening to me? As they moved through their distress, I was moved by memories of mine; a helpless new mother trying to soothe an inconsolable baby surrounded by the strange walls of a hospital room. I chose to stay and bear witness without judgement, breathing with them as they walked past for the umpteenth time.

When I first saw the mother with the child walk past me, I was a mere stranger, a background figure in the hospital waiting room. As I became a witness to the pair's distressing performance, I became entangled in their story. Their unexpected performance not only interrupted my monotonous suspension in the hospital waiting room, it moved me back to my senses and connected me with my past and present experience. It is what I refer to as kinaesthetic entanglement in this chapter.

DOI: 10.4324/9781003222484-4

A research story

Another vivid memory. It is May 2014. I am standing in the middle of a small theatre stage surveying the set up of an upcoming performance. It is a minimalist black box with 5 chairs at the back of the stage (for the performers) and enough seating for 80 viewers laid out in rows in the auditorium. I move from chair to chair nervously straightening out the rows and trying to reassure myself I am in control of the situation. Only, I am not. Because even though I have directed and curated the performance, I have no idea how it will actually unfold. The experimental and participatory dance theatre performance, in which I am about to immerse myself (and others), is entitled |mu| and is part of an interdisciplinary research project on kinaesthetic empathy.

It is this immersive experience of creative process I will explore in this chapter, through the lens of a dance theatre performance. Through performer and audience member reflections, I will reveal the dialogic interplay between mover and witness during a live performance situation. I will draw particular attention to how kinaesthesia, described also as our movement sense (Rova 2017), is experienced (by movers and witnesses) and how it informs our understanding of ourselves and others. As the writing of this chapter is situated within, and informed by, multiple socio-political, environmental and health crises, unfolding at great speed in the 21st century, I will seek to draw parallels between creativity and performance as enactive antidotes to wider issues affecting communities in a rapidly changing world.

The performance event I will discuss here was one component of the interdisciplinary research methodology I employed in my investigation of kinaesthetic empathy (Rova 2017). The research brought together Dance Movement Psychotherapy, phenomenology and cognitive neuroscience to ask: How do we feel with or understand others through our moving bodies and how does this understanding manifest verbally and non-verbally? The research concluded with the following observations: that we (human persons) have an innate capacity to experience empathy (feeling with the other) through our moving body, and this ability can be cultivated over time (Rova 2017). Essentially, not only are we innately compassionate beings but we can train ourselves to be more so. Specifically, the more connected we are with our own embodied experiences, the more compassionate and empathic we become with others. The different research methods utilised (embodied practice focus groups and brain scanning, see Rova 2017) allowed me to observe the workings of kinaesthetic empathy through unique prisms (for example, observation, reflection/introspection and embodied experience). However, it was the live performance event that brought to life the experience of witnessing another move, moving in response to another and being moved by another (physically, emotionally and mentally). Creative process opened up the space for this meeting between mover and witness to occur.

Embedded in the philosophical orientation of the research project was the idea of using the body as "a key methodological term" (Diprose & Reynolds

2008:111), since the subject of enquiry itself was no other than the process of embodiment in relationship. Allegranti (2011) describes bridging theoretical 'knowing' with embodied practice as "investigating [...] conceptual schemes or 'texts' that ontologically ground 'knowing' with/in the body" (12). The moving body was the subject, the method, the discourse and the research outcome of my investigation all at once. As such, |mu| was not a polished choreographic performance, but rather an arrangement of improvised experiential relational tasks inviting both audience members and performers to discover and create meaning together, mediated by my guiding research questions. There was an order of events, a series of tasks and opportunities for the performers and audience members to interact. After the performance, audience members and performers contributed their reflections in writing. The process-oriented nature of this performance is unique to creative artistic practices employed by arts psychotherapists and informed by a phenomenological attitudinal stance in carrying out the research project.

In all my written accounts of the work, I had been reporting with formality that this performance event contributes to the research outcomes. But in that moment standing in the middle of the black box waiting for the movers and witnesses to enter the dialogue, I felt a wave of doubt. Is experience or else 'being-in-it' a 'valid' (I sense a discomfort as I type the word) way of knowing-in-the-world? As a dancer, dance movement psychotherapist, teacher and clinician I knew this to be true. Trying to find a comfortable fit with my researcher position I was now doubting the very intention that had led me to this research path in the first place. I would later confirm my assumption that as a dancer, dance movement psychotherapist, teacher and clinician I was already engaging in research by being in and engaging others in the practice. I do not wish to be misunderstood as complacent here. Research is an intentional act. So is studying relationships in action through the transformative experience of creative embodied practice as a catalyst for change. But even the writing of the following sentence took three attempts (and still I am not satisfied with the result): "The research concluded with the following evidence, findings, possibilities observations?". I suppose what I am really asking here is: What is research for? Who is entitled/allowed/empowered to do it? And what counts as valid? Reynolds and Reason (2012) use the term 'corporeal turn' to conceptualise developing discourses of the mind and body: "[...] the corporeal turn demands that we face the challenge of considering practices and experiences that typically sit outside of reflective consciousness. Within the arts this is most explicitly manifest in the development of practice-based research" (21). As Frizell (2021) would say, the practice IS the research!

What strikes me most looking back at the above pre-show memory, from the perspective of the now post-Covid era, is the intimacy of the performance, the physicality of the relational space and the closeness experienced by all involved in the live event. During the pandemic, when people were forced to isolate, stay apart, keep their distance and avoid physical contact, the arts brought people together (even from a distance) and kept people going.

There were global virtual choirs (Camden Voices as seen in BBC London 2021), opera performances from balconies (see Italian Opera Singer serenading Florence 2021), global live art events (see Becoming Tree 2020–2021) and sharing of art work through social media (Greyson's Art Club 2020). People reached across the isolation and separation through digital and hybrid platforms to connect and co-create meaning through online gatherings and virtual performances. These were performances of survival and defiance.

What happens when we immerse ourselves in the creative process? What can we know through our moving body? How do we experience others and how are we moved by others? The next four sections, entitled respectively 'The knowing body', 'The performance journey', 'Inter-connectedness' and 'Being moved', will untangle these questions through a dialogic exploration of mover-audience reflections. Among the experiential tasks performed by the movers during the live event of |mu| was the participatory engagement of spectators as they arrived into the auditorium. Five spectators were approached at random, each by a different performer, and invited to give their response to a question written on a card posed by the researcher (for example, "what would you tell your child self if you met them today?"). During a sequence of the performance, entitled *This Story is About*, each mover embodied their response to the answer they received by an audience member as they made sense of this in the moment. The first theme emerging from the audience-performer intersubjective meeting is 'the knowing body', the realisation that through the other we can meet ourselves and vice versa.

The knowing body

I felt I could really relate to their movements

The part I feel I could comment on the most was the dancer's story around worrying. Perhaps because I too am a worrier, I felt I could really relate to their movements and that they captured them well. Interestingly the blowing they were doing is something I have done in the past as a means of trying to blow my worries away when trying to get to sleep with an overactive mind. I found it uncomfortable to watch at times as I could relate to how they felt, you know, like the thoughts were too much and were taking over. I have kept thinking about this dancer since the play so they have obviously had an impact!

(Audience member)

I had to make the experience mine

I was kind of dreading this moment. How can I re-tell someone else's story? So I read the note and noticed how the words 'hit' me; what these words mean to me and the impact they have on my body … I felt I had to make the experience mine in order to convey what this might have meant to this particular person… And suddenly I find myself doing a particular action and I try to go even deeper to this action. I struggle. I try to enlarge the feeling in myself. I notice that this helps. I even notice that my facial muscles respond to this, and here I am, I get it and lose it, I am in and out of this moment, of this feeling that is not someone else's anymore but mine…I start thinking 'am I really doing this right?', …'is my experience any close to their experience?'… It was a real relief when after the performance was finished this person came to me to express their surprise (at) how somebody that they did not even know could be in their own mind and (seemingly) feel exactly the same way they were feeling.

(Dancer)

The audience member's reflection suggests that their identification with the experience the dancer embodied facilitated their relationship with the mover and the material they were tackling whilst transposing their own layer of lived experience onto the material. Indirectly, the witness also entered into a relationship with the 'invisible' audience member who offered their story to the dancer and with me (as researcher/choreographer) who invited this dialogue through the audience participation task. This multidimensional exchange is possible because of a shared 'working kinaesthetic sense' (Paterson 2012) grounded in our bodily knowing of ourselves and in relationship with others.

The mover admits they were *dreading* the audience participation task as they were unsure whether they would be able to 're-tell' someone else's story. Notably – contrary to a conventional dance production, where the dancer may be concerned about the technical and aesthetic delivery of their performance – in '|mu|' the sense of anticipation is shared between performer and spectator as they both enter a dialogic exploration of the unknown. Through her investigation into the 'ecological aesthetics of dance', Carr (2014) explains that "(d)ance works that challenge audiences' kinaesthetic expectations may not always be easy, either to perform or watch, but may engender intercorporeal negotiations that have the potential to lead to transformation" (56). Interestingly, both the viewer and the performer became aware of, what could be described as, an 'intersubjective tension' as they entered this dynamic relationship: The audience member explains that they *found it uncomfortable to watch* at times, while the dancer speaks of *struggl(ing)* as they attempt to find a personal connection to the viewer's story. Both describe the encounter as having an *impact* on their personal experience. Paterson (2012) defines this kinaesthetic self-other reflexivity as "the proprioceptive ability to 'feel' and therefore recognise one's own body and its movements" (492). And as Jola et al (2012) suggest, dance performance engages spectators (and I would add performers as well, as evidenced by the participant reflections) on multiple levels, including perceptual, emotional, cognitive and physical.

The creative process described above reveals that the moment the story takes form (is embodied) within the intersubjective field (created by the performance event) the performer and viewer mutually recognise and co-construct each other's subjectivities. The story is now *known* by both the mover and the viewer and belongs to *both* equally *and* each separately. As Carr (2014) astutely points out:

> For the audience, engagement with the dancers' explorations of somatic experience may inform (even challenge) their own consciousness of being in the world. The potential for such responsive sensitivity may be of increasing importance to artists working in a rapidly changing social realm who aim to create work, the significance of which, while never fully shared, is available to a process of intercorporeal negotiation across difference.
>
> (57)

It may be suggested, therefore, that the kinaesthetic awareness of self-other (inter)relationships within artistic contexts may not only be of value for performers or spectators, but may also be beneficial as a social (and/or educational) intervention towards nurturing the capacity to relate to others (Aden 2014). Performing arts have the capacity to transport us to emotional landscapes, as the next two vignettes illustrate.

The performance journey

I found myself being taken on a journey

I found myself being taken on a journey through bodily reactions, emotions and memories. I felt like I was swinging between just observing and the desire to stand up, participate and explore each moment with others and by myself. In both cases, I felt there was enough space for me to stay with the performance and accept the experience fully.

(Audience member)

Audience and dancers transported elsewhere

I am also reminded of the power of an embodied dance performance where the audience and dancers are transported elsewhere during the performance. This is akin to what happens in Dance Movement Psychotherapy – the shared kinaesthetic and empathic movement experience allows clients and therapist to travel to other places and ways of being, as an exploration of the possibilities of how we might live our lives . . . The power of dance to take us to different ways of being and to then return to the here and now!

(Dancer)

The viewer relates their experience of *being taken on a journey* to their *bodily reactions, emotions and memories* triggered by the performance. Audience research has shown that "(s)pectators frequently report that even while sitting still, they feel they are participating in the dance they observe, experiencing movement sensations and related feelings and ideas" (Jola et al. 2012: 20). The audience member not only identifies a kinaesthetic response in her experience of watching the performance but also alludes to an active *desire to stand up, participate and explore*. Reason and Reynolds (2010) suggest that audience responses to dance spectatorship depend on personal experiences of dance (such as motor familiarity of movement) and other socio-cultural factors (gender, body image and fitness). It may be argued, therefore, that the experience of dance performance is situated within the intersubjective field, mutually informed by audience and performer narratives, and shaped by the cultural and environmental contexts within which they are created (Carr 2014).

The mover's reflection reveals the complexities between consciousness-world and self-other interrelationships (Carr 2014). The mover speaks from their perspective as a dancer and dance movement psychotherapist engaging in embodied explorations of kinaesthetic empathy in a live dance theatre performance context. They suggest that viewers and dancers *are transported elsewhere during the performance*. This reflection highlights the potential for the creative process to facilitate experiences of 'escapism' and self-awareness (for both movers and viewers) in the 'here and now'. Moreover, as Reason and Reynolds (2010) argue, spectator experiences of watching dance also need to be considered within the framework of 'kinaesthetic pleasure':

> The consideration of pleasure alongside that of kinesthesia allows us to recognize that for one spectator the empathetic response might be to allow themselves to be bodily carried away by an escapist flow of movement, while for another it is to feel viscerally involved in an awareness of effort, muscle, and sinew. Consideration of pleasure similarly allows us to recognize different desired self/other relations between spectator and dancer(s), which ranged from pleasure in intimacy and closeness to discomfort and displeasure in proximity and desire for aesthetic distance, including distance from one's own (imperfect) self.
>
> (72)

Despite |mu| being structured, through a sequence of performance tasks, each performance event (including the rehearsal sessions, previews and final performance) revealed new movement material and interpretations thereof. Thus, each performance became a journey (into the unknown) moulded dialogically by those present within the intersubjective field created between the performers, the audience members and the researcher/choreographer. As Sheets-Johnstone (2009) states, "intercorporeal meanings are 'etched along the lines of kinetic/tactile-kinesthetic bodies'" (231). Therefore, kinaesthetic intersubjectivity informs both individual and social discourses of self-other understandings. This self–other entanglement was also articulated as 'inter-connectedness' as seen by the following audience and mover reflections.

Inter-connectedness

Reaching wider into the world

The audience are arriving and we, the performers are with them in the space. I feel an immediate sense of intimacy with everyone who enters and settles down in their seat. I sense a mutual feeling of anticipation between them and me. From my former years of performing, I am used to a much clearer boundary between performer and audience. A deliberate disconnect even. Here, I open myself to who is entering, how they are moving and where they position themselves. As familiar bodies enter the space my small self is drawn to them and not a stranger. The part of myself that reaches wider into the world takes over and I find myself approaching the person in the room who looks the least comfortable and that I sense is looking inwards for comfort - perhaps I feel a connection? I feel (their) response to my approach and my question in my body: it has shaken them out of themself and they need time to adjust. They take a long time to respond and write a lot. I have not yet read the contents but I feel warmth and emotion moving around my body as I sense their deepening connection with the experience. This has set a tone for me now. Through this interaction I have made a connection, with the audience and with myself, which I know I must hold onto during the rest of the performance.

(Dancer)

I found myself drawn more to watching one dancer

The thing that really stood out for me was the connection I felt for a particular dancer's performance most of all. I think this might have been because they came and spoke with my partner and I. Before the performance started, they asked my partner for a suggestion which they later embodied during the performance. Because of this perhaps I found myself drawn more to watching them more than any of the other performers. Even when I became conscious of this, and tried to steer myself towards watching the others I would always find myself feeling more connected, or 'enjoying' their movement more than the other performers.

(Audience member)

The mover identified a *sense of intimacy* and *anticipation* as they witnessed the audience members take their seats in the auditorium. Perhaps it was the close proximity of the viewing area to the performance space that softened the divide between performer and spectator. Perhaps the viewers' arrival being met with the dancers' welcome into the space provided a mutual recognition of each other's humanity and vulnerability. As Carr (2014) suggests, the dancers' awareness of the presence of the spectators affects their experience of and movement within the performance space. The mover recalls 'opening' to people's movement and positioning, and *reach(ing) wider into the world* they made a connection with an audience member who seemed *the least comfortable*.

Perception seems to play a crucial role in the experience of inter-connection described by both the performer and viewer above. Sheets-Johnstone (2009) resists a separation between sensing and moving perception as she explains: "the global dynamic world I am perceiving, including the ongoing kinaesthetically felt world of my own movement, is inseparable from the kinetic world in which I am moving" (32). She goes on to suggest that movement and perception are seamlessly interwoven as "there is no 'mind-doing' that is separate from a 'body-doing'" (Sheets-Johnstone 2009: 32). In line with this perspective, and building on Gardner's distinction between kinetic and kinaesthetic perception, Victoria Gray (2012) proposes a constructive tension between the two through her investigation of empathetic experiences of stillness in performance and sculpture. Gray (2012) argues that where 'kinetic reception' involves the visual perception of movement, stillness "facilitate(s) the time and space necessary for kinaesthetic perceptions of the body to evolve between performer and spectator" (202). Challenging the conventional relationship between (the still) viewer and (the moving) performer in dance performance, Gray (2012) embodies stillness as part of her work provoking kinaesthetic responses through the shared intersubjective experiences between performer(s) and audience member(s).

The visual materiality (Sheets-Johnston 2009) of our (moving) bodies places experiences of 'seeing and been seen' at the centre of our intersubjective relationships. By *seeing* (and approaching) the audience member, and thus acknowledging their (inter)subjectivity in the moment, the mover 'shook them' into *seeing* (becoming aware of) themselves. This kinaesthetic entanglement further materialises through the movement during the dancer's embodiment of *their* (audience member's) story. The 'seer' (spectator) thus became the 'seen'. Equally, the dancer's subjectivity as the 'seeing *and* seen' mover facilitated a reciprocal and non-objectifying gaze between the performer and audience member.

Embodied performances that invite performers and spectators to (inter) actively attend to their kinaesthetic experiences of (embodying and witnessing) dance can make a valuable contribution towards wider self-other and consciousness-world understandings (Carr 2014), within clinical and social contexts. As Jola et al. (2012) suggest, "(r)ather than purely personal and private, experience is treated as socially mediated, (therefore) audiences are considered as active agents in constituting the meaning of the performance" (28). Moreover, building on Allegranti's (2011) theorisation of the moving body as autobiographical, relational and political, it may be suggested that the *context* within which our empathic responses become possible is constantly 're-configured' within the reciprocal, relational and kinaesthetic experiences we engage with. Furthermore, as creative process (and phenomenological questioning) formed the basis of this research performance, the performance context came into being moment-by-moment and was co-created by performers and audience members in this specific time and space. It is precisely because creative process enables the possibility of an 'unbroken now' that the dancers were able to revel in the moment through "an on-going flow of movement from an ever-changing kinetic world of possibilities" (Sheets-Johnstone 2009: 30). Feeling kinetically and affectively (inter)connected with another essentially allows us to 'be moved' as the final vignettes reveal below.

Being moved

By moving with others we move ourselves

Very moving, bringing me to my body. It was nice to watch, to be there but it was hard to sit and not move with the movers. (A) very sensitive piece with sincere and detailed work. We are all in one, through others we see ourselves. By moving with others we move ourselves. I am very moved.

(Audience member)

The audience has entered the relationship

The performance starts. We start to hum, meow, groan and growl. As our expressive voices begin to fill the space, I am aware of how my voice sounds in a way that I wasn't during our rehearsals. This is now a triad instead of a dyad. The audience has entered the relationship. Throughout the performance I am aware of myself, my fellow performers, the audience as a whole, and individuals within the audience. Who has a more prominent presence constantly shifts. After the performance I do not have the familiar post-show feeling of having 'conquered' a piece, a technique or an audience with the elevated rush of adrenaline which comes with it. Instead, I feel a warm satisfaction that I have joined others in a communication and connected in unexpected ways with feelings and people.

(Dancer)

The common root of the words 'moved' and 'moving', used to describe both physical movement and an emotional response, alludes to *change* as the essence of both interpretations of the word. Where physical movement denotes a change of position in time and space, 'being moved' emotionally indicates a shift in the person's affective state. The examples above expressly connect viewers' personal affective responses to their experience of watching the performance work. Through their audience research, Reason and Reynolds (2010) conclude that "(w)hether sympathetic, empathetic, or contagious, the kinesthetic experience can be described as an affect" (72). In her analysis of de Rivera's 'geometry of emotions', Sheets-Johnstone (2009) points to the tactile-kinaesthetic dynamics between movement and emotions: "all emotions resolve themselves into extensional or contractive movement, movement that goes either toward or against or away from an object, including the object that is oneself" (204). Arguably, attending to the interrelationship between movement and affective experience is one of Dance Movement Psychotherapy's most important contributions to psychotherapeutic practice and psychological understandings of embodiment.

The mover's narration brings into focus the relational and embodied exchanges happening simultaneously between performers and audience members during the dance performance. As demonstrated by the creative and phenomenological methodology used in the performance, the dancer's awareness (of themselves and others) became possible through an active recognition of the others as equal partners in the relationship. This inclusive and interactive approach, facilitating the sharing of narratives and feelings between performers and spectators, is modelled by social improvisational theatre initiatives such as Playback Theatre and August Boal's 'Forum Theatre' and 'Theatre of the Oppressed'. These examples of community performances, straddling the boundaries between artistic practice and social intervention, suggest that "the narratives we experience on a daily basis, when performed and reviewed, can provide the potential for profound change both culturally and politically" (Tucker et al. 2010: 183). These social performances invite live audiences to engage actively in the construction of personal, social and political narratives that aim to bring about personal and collective change. Another example of dance performance as social intervention and embodied activism may be seen in Allegranti's (2020) 'Moving Kinship Hubs', where bespoke dance stories for people living with young onset dementia and their families are created and performed. This activist performance practice at once offers opportunities for connection (for the people living with dementia and their loved ones), breaks down stigma (barriers of communication) and raises awareness around the lived experience of dementia with the wider public. This ethical approach of working with embodied material and performance may be of value not only within community or artistic contexts, but it may also inform/contribute to education and health policy development.

On arriving time and again

In her poem 'Sometimes' Mary Oliver (2017) implores us to "pay attention, be astonished and tell about it" (105). To pay attention to our embodied entanglements, to our connectivity with each other, the world around us, our roots, the ground beneath our feet, our happening. To be astonished by what we discover in moments of connection and integration but also (or perhaps especially) in moments of fragmentation, alienation and ambiguity. To tell (ourselves and the world) about it. Speak it, express it, move it, transform it.

Back in that hospital waiting room, in witnessing that mother and child, it was this paying of attention and my embodied response that led me to seek a window table at the hospital cafe to put some words down. The emergent story was created in the meeting point between moving bodies, the cold hospital seat, the white hospital light, the concrete floor, the stroller, the sound of the elevator arriving and departing, the stillness, the waiting, the noticing, the breathing. What will be the next kinaesthetic performance you (co)create and participate in?

Window table
hot coffee
Americano
black
no milk
no sugar
outside, the rain dances with the sunshine
"how odd"
she said,
and smiled behind her mask
hospital cafe
things swirling inside
hidden pain
unearthed
the boy in the pushchair
screaming
"mummy, mummy"
he is in distress
she is in distress
(behind her mask)
Is he in pain?
Is he afraid?
My son, my boy
memories of separation
vulnerability
I remember being pushed
along a corridor
in a wheelchair
What is it about hospitals
these places of sanctuary
yet so humiliating

Nurses on the go
no time to waste
A kindly voice in the distance asks
"Are you OK?"
"Are you sure?"
where does she find
the (com)passion?
what does she do
with the pain?
where does she put it?
a soft nest?
a warm blanket?
sometimes soft
can be painful too. . . .

References

Aden, P. (2014). Theatre education for an empathic society. In International Conference on Performing Arts in Language Learning. Research gate. Retrieved 10/08/2015, pp. 1–4.

Allegranti, B. (2011). *Embodied Performances. Sexuality, Gender, Bodies.* London/New York: Palgrave McMillan.

Allegranti, B. (2020). Dancing activism: Choreographing the material with/in dementia. In Chaiklin, S. & Wengrower, H. (eds) *Dance and Creative Process in DMT: International perspectives.* New York: Routledge, pp. 157–177.

Becoming Tree (2020). Available online. https://becomingtree.live/.

Camden Voices (2021). BBC London. https://www.youtube.com/watch?v=28mo84 ZCNUM.

Carr, J. (2014). LandMark: Dance as a site of intertwining. *Journal of Dance & Somatic Practice* 6 (1), pp. 47–59.

Diprose, R. & Reynolds, J. (eds.) (2008). *Merleau-Ponty Key Concepts.* Stocksfield: Acumen.

Frizell, C. (2021). Towards posthuman dancing subjects: A critical commentary assemblage that interrupts five published works through the lens of practice-led, new materialist research. Doctoral thesis, Goldsmiths, University of London.

Gray, V. (2012). Re-thinking stillness: Empathetic experiences of stillness in performance and sculpture. In D. Reynolds & M. Reason (eds) *Kinesthetic empathy in creative and cultural Practices,* Bristol, UK/Chicago, USA: Intellect, pp. 199–217.

Italian Opera Singer serenades Florence (2021). https://www.youtube.com/watch?v=dhTjGS3QkYE.

Jola, C., Ehrenberg, S. & Reynolds, D. (2012). The experience of watching dance: Phenomenological- neuroscience duets. *Phenomenology and the Cognitive Sciences,* 11, pp. 17–37.

Oliver, M. (2017). *Devotions.* New York: Penguin Press.

Paterson, M. (2012). Movement for movement's sake? On the relationship between kinaesthesia and aesthetics. *Essays in Philosophy* 13 (2), pp. 471–497.

Perry, G. (2020). Grayson's Art Club. Channel Four.

Reason, M. & Reynolds, D. (2010). Kinesthesia, empathy, and related pleasures: an inquiry into audience experiences of watching dance. *Dance Research Journal* 42/2 Winter, pp. 49–75.

Reason, M. & Reynolds, D. (2012). *Kinesthetic Empathy in Creative and Cultural Practices*. Bristol, UK/Chicago, USA: Intellect.

Rova, M. (2017). Embodying kinaesthetic empathy through interdisciplinary practice-based research. *The Arts in Psychotherapy* 55, pp. 164–173.

Sheets-Johnstone, M. (2009). *The corporeal turn. An interdisciplinary reader.* UK: Imprint-Academic.

Tucker, A. N., & Price, A. & Dietrich A. (2010). Reflections on performance. In Johns, C. (ed) *Guided reflection: A narrative approach to advancing professional practice* (2nd ed.). Chichester, West Sussex: Blackwell Publisher, pp. 185–202.

5 The cat, the foal and other meetings that make a difference

Posthuman research that re-animates our responsiveness to knowing and becoming

Caroline Frizell

In this chapter, I invite you to join me in thinking about post-qualitative research, inspired by new materialism and posthumanism and the exciting potential of engaging with embodied practice-led research. The writing describes the process of a research inquiry into the nature of posthuman subjectivity through diffractive analysis at the interface of Dance Movement Psychotherapy (DMP), ecopsychotherapy and critical disability studies. The focus of this chapter is on the *how* of the research (the method), rather than the *so what?* (the outcomes and conclusions) of the research. I will explore how new materialism and posthumanism trouble ideas about what it means to be human, as well as problematising dominant discourses underpinning research design, evidence and impact, moving towards research that is practised differently (Taylor, Quinn & Franklin-Phipps 2021). I take my place as a post-qualitative, practice-led researcher within the ebb and flow of an intra-acting world, within methods that enable me to remain 'responsible and responsive to the world's patternings and murmurings' (Barad 2012: 207). In terms of the immediate orientation in navigating this chapter, first, I will share my shift from qualitative to post-qualitative research, mapping out ideas from new materialism and posthumanism that have supported my approach. I will then illustrate the application of this approach through a research inquiry exploring posthuman subjectivity using diffractive analysis to move through the transversal intersections of dance, as a participatory process in psychotherapy, ecopsychotherapy, as a practice that locates the human subject within a wider ecology and critical disability studies and as a portal to non-binary practice. This writing follows the overall spirit of this edited anthology, which comprises a community of authors committed to locating the creative process at the heart of embodied research, theory and practice.

Shifting towards the post-qualitative

Over time, I have used a range of qualitative research methodologies such as case study, autoethnography and interpretive phenomenological analysis (IPA) (see, for example, Frizell 2012, 2014, 2017, 2020, 2021). With

DOI: 10.4324/9781003222484-5

hindsight, I was often left with a quiet voice of dissent, i.e. no particular methodology was a perfect fit. For example, I found IPA[1] to provide a very useful and systematic method for thinking about interview processes, drawing out themes from interview transcripts to make sense of emergent stories within wider discourses surrounding disability (Frizell 2021). However, a particular sequence of events in one of the interviews pushed the boundaries of the methodology. Thematically, this sequence of events didn't fit with the emergent narrative, yet my intuition of its significance persisted. The night before meeting one mother for an interview, I dreamt of the birth of a foal who was unlike other foals. In the perception of those who saw her, she just wasn't foal-like. I awoke with a strong sense of unease and intrigue. During the interview the following day, the mother-participant was describing how she had told her older daughter that her new sister had Down's syndrome. Her daughter, a horse enthusiast, asked if horses could have Down's syndrome. At that moment in the interview, the cat jumped onto the table, sending papers flying and using her paw to bat the microphone onto the floor, demonstrably demanding attention by nuzzling her head into my neck. It was difficult to move on.

During a thematic analysis of the interview transcripts, this moment stayed with me, yet it did not conform to the emergent themes. The sense of unease provoked by my dream began to morph into thoughts about how we create pre-existing entities in our minds about what makes a foal a foal, what makes a human a human and how Down's syndrome disrupts and disturbs what we think we know about being human. In our minds, we create Down's syndrome as a thing and those thus labelled become inscribed with the powers of its discourse. I realised that my less conscious knowing clung to a defining essence of things being represented through language. I was reminded of the film *Lobster*[2] that leads the viewer to think about 'dissolving static and binary concepts of species, gender, and the relation between them' (Barker 2018: 29). Hotel guests are sorted into pairs of perfectly suited couples. Failure to find a mate results in the relinquishing of humanhood, as individuals are transformed, somewhat brutally, into animals. As I watched, my orientation in time and space was disrupted. My sense of subjectivity grasped for meaning within the chaos. Issues of normativity bumped up against the unknown and I clung to the raft of my own subjectivity.

In watching the film, I became lost, as you, the reader, might also have begun to feel lost in this chapter. I imagine you trying to construct some conceptual scaffolding that holds these ideas together. In post-qualitative research, this has been my experience of a research process that is non-linear and demands that I tolerate not knowing where I might be taken. Do bear with me, for if we can allow ourselves to become lost, then we have an opportunity to reset our compasses.

The sequence of events that led to cat jumping on the table during that interview exposed me to a sense of the unquestioned humanist assumptions that seemed to underpin much qualitative research. The methods we use as researchers are only as potent as the kind of thinking we use to think about those methods. At about this time (of the cat jumping on the table), a chance meeting with a colleague in the university corridor (thank you Dr Jill Westwood) alerted me to new materialist perspectives and I began to follow my nose, finding my way to Barad (2003, 2007, 2012, 2014), Braidotti (1997, 2013, 2019, 2019a) and Haraway (2004, 2016) with eager enthusiasm, and, I will admit, entangled confusion. I was immediately drawn to these apparent ways of animating the world differently and rooting that animation in a bodily felt, experiential method that 'allows matter its due as an active participant in the world's becoming' (Barad 2003: 803). The notion of becoming (rather than being) is central to the post-qualitative research that I am describing. Becoming is the experiential fluidity of potential that is immersive and imminent, rendering diffusive the boundaries around a pre-existing subjective 'I'. The materiality of *body* as a dynamic active agent combines with discursive practice that creates *body-politics* as part of continuous relational movement. The notion of becoming is this experiential and intellectual edge of our creativity that infuses each moment with the potential of knowing the world differently, calling out 'in the pause that precedes each breath before a moment comes into being and the world is made again' (Barad 2007: 185).

I found myself wandering into an untamed place, where thorns and thistles know no bounds and wild orchids flourish. Where life dances as a transient butterfly in a shaft of sunlight and creeps in darkness, as a mole, in an underground world, where rhizomes wend their way through the earth, perhaps unaware of their inspiration for a Deleuze-Guattarian (Deleuze & Guattari 1987) philosophical understanding. This rhizomatic configuration, in contrast to something more linear, is key to the creation of a research assemblage that comprises the gathering of material-discursive matters around a research inquiry. The image of a rhizome conveys the complexity of a system that does not have a particular central point of reference, but rather has multiple points of emergence that can connect in multiple ways. Within a complex matrix, materiality and discourse cannot be separated and the work of Butler (2011), for example, is useful in thinking about how material human bodies become created within deeply embedded inscriptional spaces of discourse and the ways in which this entanglement of material-discursive processes cannot be neatly separated out.

New materialism has increasingly drawn interest in research (Barrett 2013; Davies 2014, 2017; Fox & Alldred 2015, 2017; MacDonald & Wiens 2019; Maclure 2013; Monforte 2018; Murris 2021; Schadler 2019; Somerville 2016; Springgay & Rotas 2015), as an ontology and epistemology that rebalances human pre-occupations and experience, which in academia has been strongly orientated around language, discourse and culture. Similarly, posthuman research (e.g., Braidotti 1997, 2013, 2019; Braidotti & Bignall 2019; van der Tuin 2019) engages transdisciplinary perspectives in knowledge production, welcoming the complex multiplicity of open-ended processes. Post-qualitative approaches to research bring our attention to the entanglement of humans in a wider ecology of matter and discourse, offering potential for new ways of perceiving and processing data (Schadler 2019).

Following my nose

As I followed my nose, I was discovering a place of radical immanence, that is 'the primacy of intelligent and self organising matter' (Braidotti 2019a: 31). St. Pierre (2021) describes a philosophy of immanence as 'concerned not with what is but what is not yet' (163). With my nose to the ground, I moved with(in) a relational tension between research and practice through which knowledge-ing, being and becoming are 'mutually implicated' (Barad 2007: 185). Barad (2007) coined the neologism 'ethic-onto-epistem-ology' (185), claiming that ethics (the application of justice), ontology (ways of being in the world) and epistemology (the theory of knowledge itself) cannot be separated from each other in the becoming of the world (Barad 2007), nor can they be separated from method itself (St. Pierre 2014). St. Pierre (2021) states that the intention of post-qualitative inquiry is to 'to experiment and create new forms of thought and life' (163), reorientating our thinking and helping us to develop the *way* in which we think about things. Haraway (2016) alerts us to the importance of the kinds of thinking that we use and the significance of the ontologies and epistemologies that underpin our thinking. She says '(i)t matters what stories make worlds and what worlds make stories' (12). In reorientating myself to, and experimenting with, new ways of thinking, this reading supported me in the challenging injustices that are perpetuated through binary thinking. These injustices are embedded in normative, dominant discourses in relation to the privileging of language and discourse over corporeality and matter, privileging ability over disability and privileging the exceptional human over the subordinated other (than human).

I was venturing into post-qualitative research, inspired by new ways of thinking about the research in which I was immersed. New materialist and posthuman discourses were particularly apt to the practice that I had developed as an eco-therapeutically orientated DMP, committed to working with differently enabled moving bodies. As I moved my way through ideas underpinning new materialism and posthumanism in relation to research and practice, I found myself simultaneously out of my depth and at the same time, I sensed that I was arriving home. Posthuman bodies, rather than being pre-existing entities, become affective flows within assemblages that include the 'human and non-human, animate and inanimate, material and abstract' (Davies 2014: 406). If research is about generating new knowledge, then it needs to enable us, as researcher-practitioners, to question the attachments that 'keep us from thinking and living differently' (Lather & St. Pierre 2013: 631).

St. Pierre (2011), who coined the term post-qualitative, challenges qualitative methodology claiming that it is grounded in a particular notion of the human, derived from the Enlightenment. This notion privileges language and cognition, perceiving the world through an anthropocentric lens

(St. Pierre 2014, 2021). Braidotti (2019) also reminds us that the term human-ity is not neutral and 'indexes access to specific powers, values and norms, privileges and entitlements, rights and visibility' (159). Social categories, such as class, race, gender, age and (dis)ability, become markers of these indices. Embedded in these categories are binary oppositions that underpin domi-nant discourses. A refusal of anthropocentrism and its inherent human excep-tionalism, leads us to contemplate more-than-human ways of knowing the world, that aligns to posthuman perspectives, as articulated, for example, by Barad (2003, 2007), Braidotti (2019), Braidotti and Bignall (2019) and Bignall and Ringney (2019).

Method as a practice

I needed a method for my research and caught myself leaning towards a method-or-no-method binary. St. Pierre (2014) states that when methodol-ogy is separated from epistemology and ontology, it is in danger of becoming formulaic, tending towards mechanised techniques (2014). She suggests that post-qualitative inquiry necessarily refuses methodological concepts, such as research design and data analysis, and is concerned rather with the philosoph-ical underpinnings of poststructuralism (St. Pierre 2021). Lather (2013) also problematises methodological inquiry and asserts that new ways of thinking can materialise as we shift from binaries into multiplicities within new mate-rialist and posthuman onto-epistemologies. However, it seemed to me that in my research it was not so much whether or not we use method, but, rather, *how* method is used. As Springgay and Truman (2017) point out, method is not a thing (a binary this, in opposition to that), but it is a practice that is experienced from the inside. This practice can shapeshift with the 'particu-lar (in)tensions' (2) that are immanent to the research. Method as a practice needs to be responsive to the unanticipated surprises that enter the research assemblage (such as foals in dreams and cats on tables), rather than particular ways of gathering and analysing data. It is the thoughts that we use to think about the research that open new directions in knowledge and that help us to imagine futures differently.

Turning point

I have led you from the disruption in the interview, to thoughts about becom-ing, to the film *Lobster*, to a collegial meeting in the corridor, to immersive reading about new materialism and posthumanism. I will now turn to a re-cent inquiry into the transdisciplinary meeting place(s) of DMP, ecopsycho-therapy and critical disability studies, with a particular focus on posthuman subjectivity. These three areas had been crucial to me as a therapist, educator and researcher. I had published widely on these areas and I wanted to deepen my understanding about their interface. I decided upon a diffractive analysis of a decade of my research publications that had explored these areas. I began to create an assemblage, seeking to optimise the potential of how subjectivity might be imagined and performed. New materialism and posthumanism offered a mode of research inquiry that twisted away from representation and interpretation, towards a curiosity about the significance and relational performativity of matter(s) (Springgay & Rotas 2015).

Creating an assemblage

Having spent some time reading around new materialism and posthumanism, I began to create a material-discursive assemblage. I selected the past publications of my own into which I wanted to inquire and began to reflect on how I had (re)presented subjectivity within the realms of DMP, ecopsychotherapy and critical disability studies. I began to keep a diary of things that seemed to matter, often guided by my intuition. If I sensed that something might be significant, I made a note of it, gradually creating a transdisciplinary symposium of things that seemed to matter. It drew on personal, professional and material encounters, makeshift artworks, dreams, improvisational movement and peer-reviewed published literature, widening the realm of what counts as knowledge. The assemblage seemed to take on a life of its own and I wasn't always sure where it was going.

Assemblages are dynamic and processual, bringing a focus to potential, that is 'of becoming rather than being' (Deleuze & Guattari 1987: 275). The component parts of the assemblage affect each other from within, creating an always-in-process production of knowledge that employs an 'affect economy' (Fox & Alldred 2015: 405), that is, the ways in which the component parts affect, and are affected by, each other, within a rhizomatic configuration. The dynamic processes within an assemblage are characterised by permeability, plurality and multiplicity with blurred, rather than definitive, boundaries between phenomena.

I was able to re-turn (in the sense of turning over) and return to (in the sense of going back to) my published research with new eyes. I edged my way through rhizomatic systems of thought that became busy with critique, whilst remaining connected to the experience of being in the world as an ethical, intra-connected, moving subject. This beginning embedded the research in the entangled nature of becoming, in a world in which the performativity of subjectivity unveils hierarchies of mattering.

Diffraction in action

I gave myself permission to play with the diffractive meeting places of DMP, ecopsychotherapy and critical disability studies, wondering how this could help me to think differently about subjectivity. Each of these areas unveils power-laden, ethical discourses that have subordinated matters of the body, privileging particular kinds of knowledge over others, privileging particular kind of bodies (and species) over others and troubling ideas about kinship.

Physicist, philosopher and feminist, Barad (2007) offers a scientific notion of diffraction as a process by which waves bend and spread as they meet an obstruction. Barad (ibid) describes how the concept of diffraction can be used as a methodological approach in research, that involves 'reading insights through one another in attending to and responding to the details and specificities of relations of difference and how they matter' (71).

It took me some time to grasp the idea of focusing on the diffractive patterns that get created in the dynamic meeting places of differences, rather than the differences themselves. I needed to make an ethico-onto-epistemological shift away from essentialist ideas about pre-existing entities, to ideas of the affective flows of emergent matter. I spent some time standing on the shoreline in a blustery wind, watching the tide come in. I became entranced by diffraction in action as I watched the bending and spreading of the waves when they encountered an obstruction. That meeting place always created something new. Davies (2021) reminds us of the unpredictable nature of diffractive research processes that can be both confronting and unsettling, but at the same time effective in stimulating new ways of thinking.

I returned (to) my published works and moved into improvisation as a part of the inquiry. I had initial thoughts about creating a site-specific performance and as the planning was underway, Covid-19 struck and my intentions were interrupted. In place of a live performance, I had an idea to work with filmed improvised movement in different landscapes (Frizell 2021a).

Practice-led post-qualitative inquiry

The process of improvisational dance as research provides an opportunity to turn towards the contingent nature of being a body, always in the process of becoming.

Barbour (2018) describes how '(e)mbodied knowledge arises in the intimate weaving of passion, experience, and varied knowledges' (241) and this embodied participatory process arises through improvisation, play and experimentation, moving into gaps and articulating new connections between ideas and experience.

Bacon (2010, 2020) emphasises the processual nature of practice as research and dance improvisation as a modality to generate knowledge is well documented (for example, Allegranti 2013; Ashley 2019; Bacon 2020; Barbour 2018; Blockmans et al. 2020; Chodorow 1999; Frizell 2020; Hayes 2013; Kramer 2015; LaMothe 2020; Manning 2012; Markula 2006; McDowall 2019; Midgelow 2021; Phelan 1993; Rova 2017; Sheets-Johnstone 2011; Stromsted 2015; Trimingham 2002). I engaged with entangled encounters that are experienced through movement in any one moment, calling upon 'spontaneity, resilience, presence, adaption, readiness, responsiveness, risk, and willingness' (Fraleigh 2019, 67).

These site-specific, filmed improvisations became central components to the inquiry assemblage. This tending toward the bodily self (Ahmed 2010;

Manning 2012) is the place of encounter in which affective flows between phenomena disrupt the notion that creativity belongs to particular individuals, leaning towards creativity as 'an affective flow between assembled bodies, things and ideas' (Fox & Alldred 2017: 86).

The new materialist and posthuman perspectives slowed me down. For example, in the making of the site-specific filmed improvisations, I found myself creating a relationship with the camera equipment and the materiality and the gaze of the camera itself, embracing the idea of the affective agency of all matter. In identifying site-specific locations, I needed to immerse myself in listening and connecting to the landscape and to somehow ask for permission to move and to film in a 'posthuman convergence' (Braidotti 2019: 153) of subjects.

I moved on the contours of the earth's body, inside the entangled matter that is earth. I would turn towards knowledge-ing as it arose from the wind, following threads of multiplicity and ambiguity. The distinction between the *me* and the *not me* (Winnicott 1971) became increasingly unclear and at the same time, the idea of subjectivity as entangled matter began to make sense. I would then replay the film, and it was often not as I had imagined it. I began to create short films, the editing of which was, itself, a process of diffraction. The site-specific filmed improvisational movement became part of the wider assemblage that enabled me to theorise further the de-centring of humans as exclusive makers of meaning and to animate the thematic threads of my existing research as a form of 'knowledge-ing . . . (as) . . . a performative enactment' (Taylor 2021: 39).[3]

Widening contexts

This research itself took place during the global pandemic, as Covid-19 highlighted and troubled binaries such as macro/micro, human/non-human, individual/society and private/public (Murris 2021), problematised notions of kinship and magnified inequalities. Public, political and academic discourses became intensified. The decade of my selected published research had spanned a period of austerity in the UK, along with an escalation of neoliberal values, particularly impacting the lives of disabled people. There had been a referendum for the UK to leave the European Union and a landslide victory for right-wing politics. Environmental consciousness regarding the ecological crisis had been catapulted into the mainstream arena. The #MeToo movement further exposed gender inequalities, and a history of racial oppression became unveiled with the Black Lives Matter (BLM) movement. This turbulent context had been an opportunity to re-orient my thinking about how identities are organised and subjectivities performed. This had significant implications for bringing a more embodied, compassionate and empathic presence into the world proactively. Ahmed (2010) suggests that the 'starting point for orientation is the point from which the world unfolds: the "here" of the body and the "where" of its dwelling' (236). This research was a timely opportunity to think about the nature of subjectivity within new materialist and posthuman modes of thinking.

Final thoughts

This chapter has offered a window into the way in which I have used post-qualitative research as a practice that teeters on the edge of spontaneous creativity, welcoming embodied processes in the exploration of becoming differently in the world. In the process of crafting the research that I describe here, I struggled with the meeting places of improvised movement, abstract concepts, theoretical perspectives, dreams and material things. In using diffractive analysis as a tool with which to return to my previously published works, I discovered the fertile interface(s) of DMP, ecopsychotherapy and critical disability studies, moving me, as curator of the research assemblage, to swim into the tide of 'a new ontological framework of becoming-subjects' (Braidotti 2019a: 33) and to shine a light on the affective movement of material-discursive bodies in relationship. My entangled position as a researcher, who was implicitly implicated in the research, oriented me towards possibilities of posthuman subjectify that emerged from my published works. In using the philosophies of new materialism and posthumanism to underpin my research, I become immersed the 'not yet' (St. Pierre 2021: 163) that was about to unfold, within an atmosphere of spontaneity, indeterminacy and multiplicity. This is the place of embodied creativity that moves away from discovering truths, to changing the way in which we can participate in the world. I hope that the ideas in this chapter will support you in creating possibilities for your own eco-ethical, practice-led research, towards animating the world differently. If you are wondering where to begin, I suggest a trip to the shoreline to watch the diffraction of the waves.

Notes

1 For details of this methodology, see Smith, Flowers and Larkin (2012).
2 *The Lobster* was directed by Yorgos Lanthimos in 2015. See: https://www.imdb.com/title/tt3464902/.
3 For the full account of this research, see Frizell (2021a).

References

Ahmed, S. (2010). Orientations matter. In Coole, D. and Frost, S. (ed.) *New materialisms: Ontology, agency & politics*. London: Duke University Press, pp. 234–257.
Allegranti, B. (2013). The politics of becoming bodies: Sex, gender and intersubjectivity in motion. *The Arts in Psychotherapy*, Vol. 40 (4), pp. 394–403.
Ashley, T. (2019). Improvisation and the earth: Dancing in the moment as ecological practice. In Midgelow, L. (ed.) *The Oxford handbook of improvisation in dance*. New York: Oxford University Press, pp. 595–610.
Bacon, J. (2020). Informed by the goddess: Explicating a processual methodology. In Williamson, A. and Sellers-Young, B. (eds.) *Spiritual herstories: Call of the soul in dance research*. Bristol: Intellect, pp. 69–87.

Bacon, J. (2010). The voice of her body: Somatic practices as a basis for creative research methodology. *Journal of Dance and Somatic Practices*, Vol. 2 (1), pp. 63–74.

Barad, K. (2014). Diffracting diffraction: Cutting together-apart. *Parallax*, Vol. 20 (3), pp. 168–187.

Barad, K. (2012). On touching—the inhuman that therefore I am. *Differences*, December, Vol. 23 (3), pp. 206–223.

Barad, K. (2007). *Meeting the universe halfway: Quantum physics and the entanglement of matter and meaning.* London: Duke University Press.

Barad, K. (2003). Posthumanist performativity: Toward an understanding of how matter comes to matter. *Signs*, Vol. 28 (3), Gender and Science: New Issues (Spring), pp. 801–831.

Barbour, K. (2018). Dancing epistemology. Situating feminist analysis. In Fraleigh, S. (ed.) *Back to the dance itself: Phenomenologies of the body in performance.* CA: Illinois, pp. 233–246.

Barker, J. (2018). A Horse is a horse, of course, of course: Animality, transitivity, and the double take. *Somatechnics*, 8 (1), pp. 27–47.

Barrett, E. (2013). Materiality, affect, and the aesthetic image. In Barrett, E. and Bolt, B. (eds.) *Carnal knowledge: Towards a 'new materialism' through the arts.* London: I.B. Tauris & Co Ltd, pp. 63–72.

Blockmans, I., De Schauwer, E., Van Hove, G. and Enzlin, P. (2020). Retouching and revisiting the strangers within: An exploration journey on the waves of meaning and matter in dance. *Qualitative Inquiry*, Vol. 26 (7), pp. 733–742.

Bignall, S. and Ringney, D. (2019). Indigeneity, posthumanism and nomad thought: Transforming colonial ecologies. In Braidotti, R. and Bignall, S. (eds.) *Posthuman ecologies: Complexity and process after Deleuze.* Maryland: Rowman & Littlefield International Ltd. Pp. 159–182.

Braidotti, R. (2019a). A theoretical framework for the critical posthumanities. *Theory, Culture & Society*, Vol. 36 (6), pp. 31–61.

Braidotti, R. (2019). *Posthuman knowledge.* Cambridge: Polity Press.

Braidotti, R. (2013). *The posthuman.* Cambridge: Polity.

Braidotti, R. (1997). Meta(l)morphoses. *Theory, Culture and Society*, Vol. 14 (2), pp. 67–80.

Braidotti, R. and Bignall, S. (eds.) (2019). *Posthuman ecologies: Complexity and process after Deleuze.* Maryland: Rowman & Littlefield International Ltd.

Butler, J. (2011). *Bodies that matter.* New York: Routledge.

Chodorow, J. (1999). Dance therapy and the transcendent function. In Pallaro, P. (ed.) *Authentic movement: Essays by Mary Starks Whitehouse, Janet Adler and Joan Chodorow.* London: Jessica Kingsley, pp. 236–252.

Davies, B. (2021). *Entanglement in the world's becoming and the doing of new materialist Inquiry.* New York: Routledge.

Davies, B. (2017). Animating ancestors: From representation to diffraction. *Qualitative Inquiry*, 23 (4), pp. 267–275.

Davies, B. (2014). Reading anger in early childhood intra-actions: A diffractive analysis. *Qualitative Inquiry*, Vol. 20 (6), pp. 734–741.

Deleuze, G. and Guattari, F. (1987). *A thousand plateaus: Capitalism and schizophrenia.* London: Continuum.

Fox, N. and Alldred, P. (2017). *Sociology and the new materialism.* London: Sage.

Fox, N. and Alldred, P. (2015). New materialist social inquiry: Designs, methods and the research-Assemblage. *International Journal of Social Research Methodology*, Vol. 18 (4), pp. 399–414.

Fraleigh, S. (2019). A philosophy of the improvisational body. In Midgelow, L. (ed.) *The Oxford handbook of improvisation in dance*. New York: Oxford University Press, pp. 65–88.

Frizell, C. (2021a). Towards posthuman dancing subjects: A critical commentary assemblage that interrupts five published works through the lens of practice-led, new materialist research. Goldsmiths, University of London: unpublished thesis.

Frizell, C. (2021). Learning disability imagined differently: An evaluation of interviews with parents about discovering that their child has down's syndrome. *Disability & Society*, Vol. 36 (10), pp. 1574–1593.

Frizell, C. (2020). Reclaiming our innate vitality: Bringing embodied narratives to life through dance movement psychotherapy. In Williamson, A. and Sellers-Young, B. (eds.) *Spiritual herstories: Call of the soul in dance research*. Bristol: Intellect, pp. 207–220.

Frizell, C. (2017). Entering the world: Dance movement psychotherapy and the complexity of beginnings with learning disabled clients. In Unkovich, G., Buttee, C. and Butler, J. (eds.) *Dance movement psychotherapy with people with learning disabilities: Out of the shadows, into the light*. Abingdon: Routledge, pp. 9–21.

Frizell, C. (2014). Discovering the language of the ecological body. *Self and Society: An International Journal for Humanistic Psychology*, Vol. 41 (4), pp. 15–21.

Frizell, C. (2012). Embodiment and the supervisory task. *Body, Movement and Dance in Psychotherapy: An International Journal for Theory, Research and Practice*, Vol. 7 (4), pp. 293–304.

Haraway, D. (2016). *Staying with the trouble*. London: Duke University Press.

Haraway, D. (2004). Modest_Witness@Second_Millennium. In Haraway, D. (ed.) *The Haraway reader*. New York: Routledge, pp. 223–250.

Hayes, J. (2013). *Soul and spirit in dance movement psychotherapy: A transpersonal approach*. London: Jessica Kingsley.

Kramer, P. (2015). *Dancing materiality: A study of agency and confederations in contemporary outdoor dance practices*. Coventry University: Unpublished PhD Thesis.

LaMothe, K. (2020). Writing why we dance: The predicament, pitfalls, potential and promise of writing about dance and spirituality. In Williamson, A. and Sellers-Young, B. (eds.) *Spiritual herstories: Call of the soul in dance research*. Bristol: Intellect, pp. 393–413.

Lather, P. (2013). Methodology-21: What do we do in the afterward? *International Journal of Qualitative Studies in Education*, Vol. 26 (6), 634–645.

Lather, P. and St. Pierre, E. (2013). Post-qualitative research. *International Journal of Qualitative Studies in Education*, Vol. 26 (6), pp. 629–633.

MacDonald, S. and Wiens, B. (2019). Mobilizing the "Multimangle": Why new materialist research methods in public participatory art matter. *Leisure Sciences*, Vol. 41 (5), pp. 366–384.

MacLure, M. (2013). Researching without representation? Language and materiality in post-qualitative methodology. *International Journal of Qualitative Studies in Education*, Vol. 26 (6), pp. 658–667.

Manning, E. (2012). *Always more than one: Individuation's dance*. Durham: Duke University Press.

Markula, P. (2006). The dancing body without organs Deleuze, femininity, and performing research. *Qualitative Inquiry*, Vol. 12 (1), February, pp. 3–27.

McDowall, L. (2019). Exploring uncertainties of language in dance Improvisation. In Midgelow, L. (ed.) *The Oxford handbook of improvisation in dance*. New York: Oxford University Press, pp. 185–206.

Monforte, J. (2018). What is new in new materialism for a newcomer? *Qualitative Research in Sport, Exercise and Health*, Vol. 10 (3), pp. 378–390.

Midgelow, V. (2021). Practice-as-research. In Dodds, S. (ed.) *The Bloomsbury companion to dance studies.* London: Bloomsbury, pp. 111–144.

Murris, K. (2021). Making kin: Postqualitative, new materialist and posthumanist research. In Murris, K. (ed.) *Navigating the post qualitative new materialist and critical posthumanist terrain across disciplines: An introductory guide.* London: Routledge, pp. 1–21.

Phelan, P. (1993). *Unmarked.* London: Routledge.

Rova, M. (2017). Embodying kinaesthetic empathy through interdisciplinary practice-based research. *The Arts in Psychotherapy*, Vol. 55, pp. 164–173.

Schadler, C. (2019). Enactments of materialist ethnography: Methodological framework and research processes. *Qualitative Research*, Vol. 19 (2), pp. 215–230.

Sheets-Johnstone, M. (2011). *The primacy of movement.* Philadelphia: John Benjamins Pub. Co.

Springgay, S. and Rotas, N. (2015). How do you make a classroom operate like a work of art? Deleuzeguattarian methodologies of research-creation. *International Journal of Qualitative Studies in Education*, Vol. 28 (5), pp. 552–572.

Springgay, S. and Truman, S. (2017). On the need for methods beyond proceduralism: Speculative middles. In *Tensions, and Response-ability in Research. Qualitative Inquiry*, Vol. 1 (12), pp. 203–214.

Stromsted, T. (2015). Authentic movement and the evolution of soul's body® work. *Journal of Dance & Somatic Practices*, Vol. 7 (2), pp. 339–357.

St. Pierre, E. (2021). Why post qualitative inquiry? *Qualitative Inquiry*, Vol. 27 (2), pp. 163–166.

St. Pierre, E. (2014). A brief and personal history of post qualitative research toward "Post Inquiry". *Journal of Curriculum Theorizing*, Vol. 30 (2), pp. 2–19.

St. Pierre, E.A. (2011). Post qualitative research: The critique and the coming after. In Denzin, N. and Lincoln, Y. (eds.) *Sage handbook of qualitative inquiry* (4th ed.), Los Angeles, CA: Sage, pp. 611–635.

Taylor, C. (2021). Knowledge matters: Five propositions concerning the reconceptualisation of knowledge in feminist new materialist, posthumanist, postqualitative approaches. In Murris, K. (ed.) *Navigating the post qualitative new materialist and critical posthumanist terrain across disciplines: An introductory guide.* London: Routledge, pp. 22–42.

Taylor, C., Quinn, J. and Franklin-Phipps, A. (2021). Rethinking research 'use': Reframing impact, engagement and activism with feminist new materialist, posthumanist and postqualitative research. In Murris, K. (ed.) *Navigating the post qualitative new materialist and critical posthumanist terrain across disciplines: An introductory guide.* London: Routledge, pp. 169–189.

Trimingham, M. (2002). A methodology for practice as research. *Studies in Theatre and Performance*, Vol. 22 (1), pp. 54–60.

van der Tuin, I. (2019). Deleuze and diffraction. In Braidotti, R. and Bignall, S. (eds.) *Posthuman ecologies: Complexity and process after Deleuze.* Maryland: Rowman & Littlefield International Ltd. pp. 1–16.

Winnicott, D.W. (1971). *Playing and Reality.* London: Tavistock.

6 *Offerings* tells the stories of our lives in movement

Sarah Black-Frizell and Angela Pierre Louis

Sarah and Angie are dance artists and scholars based in Liverpool, and our practices engage with site, improvisation, ethics and the maternal. *Offerings* began during the UK Lockdown (2020), and it is ongoing practice as research. We called upon additional disciplines outside of performance-related areas in order to cultivate insights into maternal states and home during the pandemic. We wanted to develop awareness, understanding and different disciplines, resulting in the methodology becoming transdisciplinary (Kershaw & Nicholson 2011). This methodology developed out of our commitments to flexibility, rigour and support to address the complexity of the ways in which notions of home and the maternal have been highlighted by the pandemic. We have created *Offerings* to bring these three areas together via feminist ethics and address the ethical implications of such work. Overall, this chapter reveals a reflective account of working in the home and testifies to the intimate nature, importance and value of self as researcher.

Offerings is a practice which exposes for interrogation and critical understanding the ontology of mothering and home life in pandemic conditions. We propose *Offerings* as a methodology which is transferable and can be explored by artists interested in this kind of work, maternal studies, interdisciplinary process and sited practices. Our use throughout, both of the term 'we' and our first names, makes explicit the origins of this jointly authored reflection in shared experiences of developing methodology and creative practice. Our offerings is deliberately integrated in the text. This approach and level of informality is fuelled by our desire to echo the contingent development of the practice and unformulaic modality of the *Offerings*.

This approach, along with including lists of keywords before each section, responds to dance scholarship and writing, especially that of Miranda Tufnell and Chris Crickmay (1990, 2004) (Figures 6.1–6.3).

DOI: 10.4324/9781003222484-6

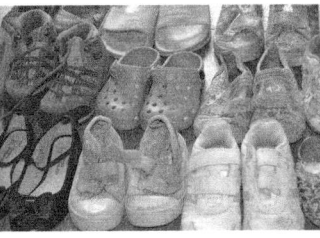 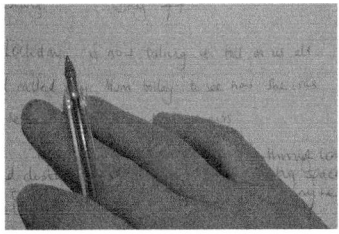 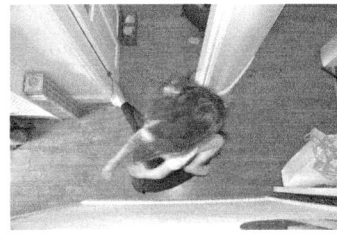

Figure 6.1   *Figure 6.2*   *Figure 6.3*

Composite Images of home. Photographs by the authors.

Pandemic   home   movement   narratives   maternal

      Sarah
          hanging
             in door
                frame
      wrapping of gentle arms

We conceptualise *Offerings* as a thing offered, a contribution towards the development of a creative practice. An *Offering* is a vessel that takes the form of a repository of information, experience and understanding of personal reflections. *Offerings* unveils an intimate, corporeal and textual exploration of mothering at home through the pandemic, and the ethical implications we encountered. When creating an *Offering*, a series of layers is formed; the practice, reflexive accounts of the experience of making the practice, and our experience of writing the reflexive accounts, all of which feature here. All *Offerings* contribute to the creation of a whole process and may include movement explorations, images, anecdotal text, scores and letters, offered between two (or more) people as part of an ongoing process in a creative practice. *Offerings* are malleable enough to accommodate and adapt to the varying needs and demands of working lives and family structure. The act of reflexive writing is a sited practice in itself, in which we aim to balance intimate details of our lives and creative practice. We borrow from auto-ethnographic practices, so as to explore personal experience, and narratives of family, as relational and

reflexive writing practice. Researching family and everyday events privileges subjectivity and emotionality; therefore, similar to an auto-ethnographic approach, our position as mother/artist/researcher influences our
Offerings (Bochner & Ellis 2000) (Table 6.1).

Table 6.1 Power consent negotiate family

Angie	Sarah
I seek my family's consent to explore interactions, conversations and exchanges that move into my own physical narratives. These shift from exploring experiences on an individual basis to whole family dynamics. Environment, space and time is always considered; when I work I bring my attention to who is at home, what is occurring in their lives and primarily their well-being. As young adult men they are supportive of my play and explorations, but explicitly resistant to physical interaction and visual documentation.	I incorporate my children in the art making, and our family home as the place of engagement. My concern when researching with my children is to enable them explicitly to consent, and their willing involvement in creative work. When the creative focus is on motherhood, my children are free to come and go; when the focus is on the children, it becomes our work, the nature of consent is different. This way of approaching consent and power emphasises my duty of care and what I believe to be in the best interests of the child (Alderson, 2001). I explore and establish parameters of consent between the mother and child as an extension of my own mothering practice.

Letter to Sarah Day 13
The children are occupied. So now is my time
We have been in the house for two weeks
I had no need to wait for something to emerge but rather I had to shift through the
many sensations and memory's that lay, rested and waited within me . . . my mind
invited my body to move and I followed . . .

Sensation   **reciprocity**   **memory**   **wait**

solace

Offerings debate our identities, locations and concerns as mothers during the
pandemic. As a methodology, *Offerings* created a space for us as mothers and
artists to retreat to, a creative space within isolation. Here, we could explore
the complexities of living through a pandemic and share our lived realities.
In *this* space, we created *Offerings*, read and responded to *Offerings* as acts of
kindness and support, inspirations and provocations, and later as catalysts for
discussion and reflection.

Offerings started at a time of great uncertainty and fear, and as such
reciprocity and care became significant rather than expectation. This was
important to us as we felt isolated in our home spaces and the challenge
of parenting through the pandemic was complex and messy. Through
Offerings, we found solace and a way of communicating our inner voices,

but without pressure or expectation. The methodological structure was the sending and receiving of an *Offering*; notions of care, creativity and openness came from spending time absorbing the materials, and thinking: Where we might go next? By this we mean there was no onus on the recipient to respond in any way, or at all. In this way, *Offerings* was a carefully curated collection of artefacts which could invite and inspire ongoing inquiry in each other's homes. *Offerings* were gifted without prior expectation of how they would be received, or what might be taken, and potentially explored in the next *Offering*.

Gaps between sending and receiving *Offerings* were dictated by the rhythms of our lives, so it was a surprise when they did come, either by mail or inbox. They were accepted without burden, and enabled perspectives on the thematic content and lived context of the pandemic, maternal and home, to be communicated and considered. This process was like a conversation and like most conversations there were pauses and interruptions, but mainly the gentle development of ideas, to which we returned, added to, supported and shaped (Table 6.2).

Table 6.2 An insight into process

Angie	Sarah
I find a space where I am alone Time to let go, declutter, I allow experiences to emerge. I begin to shift between stillness and moving, sensation and awareness.	*I write to understand daily events, emotions. I find spaces that speak to the way I am feeling as a way to process happenings in the home.*
How am I feeling? Internalising the encounters and challenges, unfinished conversations, as I move, I begin to unravel and enliven this.	*The writing maybe words, ideas, feelings, dreams. I leave the words for a day or two, allowing them to absorbed by the flesh and deeper still into my body.*
I do not continually move, I sit, reflect, return and move.	*I take this material into a space where I let the ingredients of the words, busyness of the house, inform a movement exploration. I pay particular attention to the home space; hand prints, walls, clutter and to the sounds; children, TV, banging and to the smells of my immediacy.*

Offerings – *a collection of text and images*

Sarah offering *pressure*

This *Offering* is an embodied response to a series of anecdotal writing passages during the first Lockdown. I chose to develop a visual language to

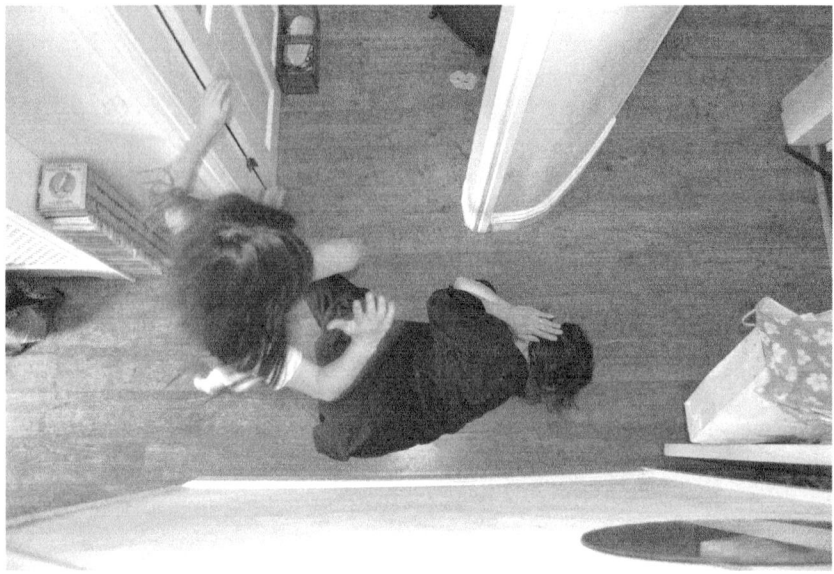

Figure 6.4 Isabel jumping over Sarah. Photograph by the authors.

voice private and intimate experiences, realised as a duet between mother and daughter that reveals this relationship as complex, changing and replete with ethical questions (Baraitser 2009) (Figure 6.4).

Day 30 Pressure

I am failing as a mother, and as a teacher of my children, I am trying to be all of these things.
I place my hand gently on the wall, a boundary between us
I send weight down through my arm into my hand
I am met with resistance, I, we cannot escape
Physical resistance of brick and mortar
Playful resistance of children.

Sarah's reflection

Revisiting where I wrote the passages, sitting on the stairs, in the hallway. I read the anecdotal writing and begin to move. '*I place my hand gently on the wall, a boundary between us*' gave rise to short improvisations. I focus on the borders, the brick and mortar confining me, and push against it with my flesh, exploring my internal landscape, blocked, resistant. This spatial relationship raises questions and feelings of isolation I am experiencing due to the pandemic and this interests me. I bring together ideas from the text; the notion of days and isolation, borders and resistance and 'I send weight down through my arm into my hand, I am met with resistance' the floor. I scale the small space around me, keeping in contact with my domestic surroundings. This begins as a solo and shortly becomes a duet. Isabel joins with me, she playfully interrupts my focus with her energy and this draws my attention to her. 'Playful resistance of children'.

Interruption is a defining maternal experience; Baraitser (2009) questions whether this fundamentally changes a mother's experience of being. In one way, interruption or disruption makes it difficult to exist in the domain of one's own reflective maternal space of experience (Baraitser 2009). The child in her moment of interruption, preventing the mother from continuing in her solo exploration, provides an opening to create something new. This duet lifted me from my solo of 'I, we cannot escape'. This shifted my attention to a moment of becoming with my child; movement as transcendence.

Moving   excavate

banal home

complexities   daily

Diary Day 117

I feel smaller, I could descend upon and into myself, folding inward, turning upon myself. Inward smaller and smaller, does anyone see me, hear me. Tighter and tighter, softly and gently disappearing into myself.

Moving is a significant aspect of *Offerings* as for us it provides a means to evacuate experience and locate our inner voices (Tuffnell & Crickmay 1990). Developing an extended sited movement practice in the home during the pandemic presented a series of possibilities and challenges. Confined by our immediate surroundings, we explored the mundane banality, interruption from children, uncertainty, arguments and tension of daily life and reconfigured this into creative practice. The pandemic gave rise to a particular palate of creativity, which was explored as a provocation or an impulse to move and move in a particular way. The *Offerings* were solo endeavours on the surface, as we were moving in our home environments, but we were connected through the offering of the Other. By working in this way, we opened the private sphere of our homes, reclaiming and re-figuring them to reveal care and labour, sharing our homes as meaningful places, holding significance of and for family (Blunt & Dowling 2006; Blunt & Varley 2004).

Diary Day 87

I've walked through the house counting the rooms, noticing the hand marks, toy marks, food splatters on the walls, the jobs that I would do, but I don't have the energy for.

Isabel is my shadow, she follows me from room to room, our personal dance. I find ways to entertain her, but the games only last minutes and we have hours to kill. If we were to do this in the winter, it would be a different experience. The yard, as small as it is, provides some outside space where we watch the clouds pass over head. There is an absence of planes, the skies are ringing with the sound of bird song, which in an inner-city area is a beautiful thing, bringing nature closer to us, replacing the sound of industry.

She takes my hand.

There is solace in the embrace of one small hand clasping onto mine Where do I end and she begins.

I can see it in her eyes; and feel it in her body when I hold her. Tension and fear melts away, but rises back up again.

She asks will we always have to live in lockdown.
Will we always be at home.

Offerings – *a collection of text and images*

Angie offering *boundaries*

Connectivity to Sarah's *Offering* Pressure

The image of the mother suspended in the doorway, looking to her child, distilled in me the permission/courage to explore my own maternal narrative.

Response to Sarah's offering

On opening Sarah's *Offering*, my attention was drawn directly to the suspended image of her at a doorframe in her home, of what appeared to be a living room. Her body positioned/hung, not weighted, but rather elevated and powerful. Was she a viewer, witnessing her home and family within it? I noticed my own need and desire to have this close and playful connection with the boys. I sensed Sarah was coping, the strength in her back demonstrated her ability to balance all the stuff that needed to be sorted, completed, the multiple needs and expectations required especially during the lockdown of being a mother, teacher (Figure 6.5).

At first, I could not respond, move, or write but it did provoke me to allow myself time and space to consider how full and busy, bitty, juggling my life felt, there was always so much to do (what was there to do!!!). I returned to the image of Sarah at her doorway defining the frame, a boundary between.

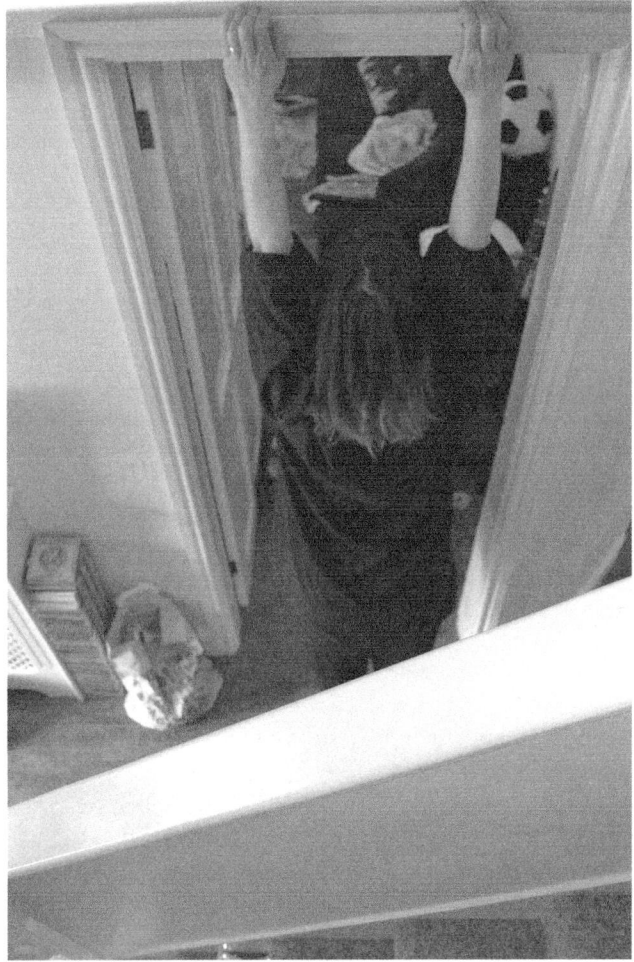

Figure 6.5 Sarah hanging from door frame. Photograph by the authors.

I thought of Gabe……. I miss touch, the wrapping of gentle arms, hanging out and connection beyond functional existence…….. How at times did I feel distant from my family when we are so close geographically, passing between doorways and landings?

Angie offering *boundaries*

A collection of written passages, images from movement scores.

Day 120 Boundaries
Boundaries . . . is this actually a space to consider, breathe, take stock. . .
.

I wonder (now, at this moment/BEFORE, a while ago) if the boundaries are a
gift, offer space, freedom a release.
A feeling draws me to the corners of a room where I am able to settle, seated on the
floor. Familiar objects close to me that do not move, stay the same, whereby I under-
stand and acknowledge their function and purpose
Why do I feel unable to cope?
Is this ok
I notice myself hovering, hanging around.

Angie's reflection

A lament exploring my feeling of being invisible and navigating the fear I had held on to one son too tightly, whilst letting the other go…. Feeling imbalanced about the boys led me to moving in the spaces between their bedrooms.

Moving my attention was in a sense, another way of 'thinking' but one that produces ideas impossible to conceive in stillness (De Spain 2003: 27).

Doors as metaphors.

I was drawn to the new boundaries created by my sons during the pandemic, and as they shifted away from me, as our conversations diminished the desire to move increased, a process of moving and re-moving to focus on how I was feeling. By moving I was able to process the clutter and confusion to find some clarity.

Ethical   home   interrelational   care   support

The significance for us is our understanding that ethics is both a methodological concern and a key dimension of practice. We consider how care and ethics are positioned through the relational work we do as mothers, the care of our relationship with each other and the process in curating the content of the *Offerings*.

The development of our ethical awareness through the doing has thereby led to a politics that allows for ways of creating, facilitating and speaking through our practice. Therefore, ethics becomes a way of responding to our environment – the home – which unearths a deep connection between ethos and lived, everyday experience.

In our *Offerings*, our ethical engagement is with the particularities of the relationship between mother and child, itself a potential paradigm for moral interaction (Baraitser 2009). We focus on thinking maternally, experiencing motherhood as a practice encompassing the ways we approach the daily tasks of mothering, our attitude to care and to art making. Through the pandemic, a particular thoughtfulness has emerged through our mothering, which, in itself, engenders ethical practice.

Diary Day 239
Young arms warm me, still me, soothe me, I pause.

In our *Offerings*, we express through our creative practice the difficulties and challenges during the day-to-day involvement of **mothering** and **maintenance** of daily life. Like Tyler and Baraitser, we suggest that the artistic processes of the **mother–artist** are not 'distinct for the work of the artist, but are on the contrary **enabling life and art'** (Tyler & Baraitser 2013: 3).

As with ethically focused or driven artistic work, we encountered implications and issues along our journey. One of our aims was to resist finding solutions to our ethical encounters and to develop a series of principles which inform our actions. We captured our intentions using documentation modes sensitive to our circumstances (Black-Frizell 2019). This led to recognising the ways we can make performance together in such turbulent times with the intention to ultimately enhance our lived experience, verifying that 'the manner in which we achieve our transforming and transformative goals is as important as the resultant work that we may ultimately present' (Bannon 2018 cited in Midgelow 2019: 1). We were learning from our human entanglements, the unpredictable and shifting relationships with self, other and family – ethics in practice. Whilst we could not share physical space, we shared a conceptual/maternal space. Through this emerging awareness, we found value in acknowledging our needs individually and collectively. Through the doing of the *Offerings*, we lived the experience of researching in this way, and felt its consequences, which we could share through our reflexive accounts.

Offerings – *a collection of text and images*

Sarah offering – *ship in the ocean*

Connectivity to Angie's *Offering* Boundaries
If boundaries are a gift? I connect with the ways Angie is working through her maternal layers of guilt and pain, trying to rationalize the ways her sons are moving away from her..
Her body framed between the pathway of the doors.

Response to Angie's offering

> *The frustrating thing was I could not hold Angie, I watched silently, and connected with the Mother moving through her space with so much care. addressing the*

boundaries-obstacles in her way. Her honesty in the text provides me with a connection I feel I need with other mothers.
The mother teetering on the edge, holding her breath silently framed.
Defining her space, holding tight.
I wanted to hold her, embrace and dance with her.
I find connection with Angie, I move to the banister and look down. I am not sure how this will manifest in my body, but I take forward the feeling of defining my space, an off-balance precarious space. I can't move yet. So, I write.

Sarah offering – *ship in the ocean*

I lost track of the days, I only know where I am with my daily writing, photographs and notes to guide me.

I have watched the world unravel in many complicated and violent ways, the virus is holding the world in panic.

In my home we keep going, the days are long, the sun rises early and sets late. There are long extended periods of quiet, the children sit in the yard picking at stones and ants.

Some days I sit on the step, and listen to their voices, loud.

Rebounding off walls.

Turning corners and following me.

They need a different kind of parenting now, out of their school routine and engulfed by their home-ness, they need reassurance, mothering with a different notion of care, a form of navigation through time and into unsafe waters. Drip-feeding information to keep them safe. But I don't feel safe.

I drift into the darker side of my mind… of mothering….

Reflection

I take up Angie's position in her film. I drift to the complex times of mothering through the pandemic and my desire to share this with Angie.

I wait, I am overcome with feelings of fear for the children, the complexity of negotiating this time. Imogen Tyler says, 'lived maternal experience remains, in a fundamental sense, unspeakable' (Tyler in Baraitser 2013: 24). So, I move slowly so as to steady my mind and body, to take stock.

I have found moving in the home so difficult situated in daily life of the pandemic. Moving is such an investment, and this is exasperated whilst trying to perform daily life duties. I am trying to maintain material and emotional conditions of myself and the children. Baraitser (2009) reveals hidden time that we experience in the day-to-day durational activities in the maintenance of daily life.

I am consumed with the darker side of mothering through the pandemic, my fears exasperated. My desire was to share with Angie occurrences that I felt she had in common. As Andrea O' Reilly (2007) states:

> I believe increasingly that only the willingness to share private and some-times painful experiences can enable a woman to create a collective de-scription of the world which will be truly yours.
>
> (7)

Conclusion

Diary Day 105
Walk, walking together
What do people see when they look in our windows

Offerings is an ongoing journey, and we have paused to write this chapter and share our thoughts, experiences and creative practice so far....

No-expectations initiated a different way of working where our focus was not solely on the production of art-making materials but on acknowl-edging what we needed as mothers/artists during that unprecedented time. So much of *Offerings* developed in response to the prevailing global climate and the complex demands of how we managed at home with our families. By working in this way, we created a sensitive approach where the opportunity to offer and respond artistically testified to the intimacy, importance of self as research and therefore infused our lives with a new political sensitivity.

Offerings embodied and questioned a set of aesthetic principles and creative approaches, which resulted in certain artistic signatures which evolved as we lived through the pandemic, alongside family. We are not abandoning aesthetic concerns, but emphasising our personal experiences through careful composition and a home-baked style (Lippard 1984).

Offering our practice back and forth gave us the opportunity to learn/ know more about each other, and share this time in a unique way. One of our questions, moving onto the next part of this journey, is one concerned with our children. Was part of the reason to do this to share the darker side of mothering through a pandemic with our children – a documenta-tion of how we really felt, an account of our daily existence and the fear we felt for our children living through these times? What would be the ethical considerations of sharing this with our children, what would they learn.......

Letter to Angie Day 20
It is Saturday morning, but the days all feed into one now.

I must call my mum to see how she is.
The children are gravitating to their devices more, as they can chat with their
friends, they drift away to their rooms. I can hear their voices, lots of laughter. Will
this be it for them, a mediated life, with no touch, no person-to-person interaction.
How will we live a life without touch, empty hands?
I walked to a local shop. I saw a mother with her children in the queue, one child
obediently holds onto the mother's hand, and a baby holding a mask, sucking the
corner of it.
No joy, no chatting,
I see a man with a homemade mask.

We would like to share the experience of watching and engaging in our work.

https://pierrea67.wixsite.com/homebaked.

References

Bannon, F. (2018). *Considering ethics, dance, theatre and performance.* Leeds, UK: Palgrave MacMillan.

Baraitser, L. (2009). *Maternal encounters: The ethics of interruption.* London: Taylor & Francis.

Baraitser, L. & Segal, L. (2009). Lynne Segal in conversation with Lisa Baraitser. *Studies in the Maternal*, 1(1), pp. 1–19.

Baraitser, L. & Spigel, S. (2009). Editorial: Mapping maternal subjectivities, identities and ethics. *Studies in the Maternal*, 1(1), p. 1.

Baraitser, L. & Tyler, I. (2013). Private view, public birth: Making feminist sense of the new visual culture of childbirth. *Studies in the Maternal*, 5(2), pp. 1–27.

Black-Frizell, S. (2019). Mother as curator: Ethical encounters in art making with children. *Conceicao Conception*, 8(2), pp. 166–185.

Blunt, A. & Dowling, R. (2006). *Home (key ideas in geography).* Abingdon: Routledge.

Blunt, A. & Varley, A. (2004). Geographies of home. Cultural Geographies. [Online] Available at: https://doi.org/10.1191/1474474004eu289xx [Accessed: 15th January 2020].

Bochner, P. & Ellis, C. (2000). Autoethnography, personal, narrative, reflexivity, researcher as subject. In Denzin, N. K. & Lincoln, Y.S. (eds.), *Sage handbook of qualitative research.* California: Sage Publications, pp. 733–762.

De Spain, K. (2003). The cutting edge of awareness: Reports from the inside of improvisation. In Albright, A.C., & Gere, D. (eds.), *Taken by surprise: A dance improvisation reader.* Middletown, CT: Wesleyan University Press, pp. 27–40.

Kershaw, B. (2011). Practice as research: Transdisciplinary innovation in action. In Kershaw, B. & Nicholson, H. (eds.), *Research methods in theatre and performance (research methods for the arts and humanities).* Edinburgh: Edinburgh University Press, pp. 63–86.

Lippard, L.R. (1984). Activating activist art: CIRCA [Online]. Available at: https://doi.org/10.2307/25556892. [Accessed: 10th December 2020].

Mideglow, V. (2019). Editorial: Ethics and performance. *Conceicao Conception*, 8 (2), pp. 1–6.

O'Reilly, A. (2007). *Maternal theory essential readings.* Toronto: Demeter Press.

Tufnell, M. & Crickmay, C. (1990). *Body space image: Notes towards improvisation and performance* (3rd ed). London: Dance Books.

Tufnell, M. & Crickmay, C. (2004). *A widening field: Journeys in body and imagination.* London: Dance Books.

Tyler, I. & Baraitser, L. (2013). Private view, public birth: Making feminist sense of the new visual culture of childbirth. *Studies in the Maternal,* 5(2), pp. 1–27.

7 Lives transformed through dance

The art of dance as a catalyst for personal transformation

Ellen Steinmüller

Introduction

Underlying all of my professional practice is the profound belief in the transformative power of dance. This prevails in my performance work as a contemporary dancer, in the therapeutic space with clients as a Dance Movement Psychotherapist and in the rehearsal studio with marginalised and vulnerable populations as a Community Dance artist and choreographer. Many times over, I had the great privilege to facilitate a process of discovery and realisation of potential, to light little sparks of confidence and to sow seeds of self-belief. Accompanying and supporting others in their journeys of self-realisation is what motivates me and what makes my work so rewarding. My chapter thus investigates the core question of how dance can serve 'as a powerful catalyst' (Annable-Coop 2016: 14) for these journeys of personal transformation and proposes that this is realised by empowering individuals to shape their sense of self actively and creatively.

In no other context have I had the opportunity to witness the transformative potential of the art of dance so fully realised in embodied action than in my work with the pioneering dance development company *Dance United*. The company's methodology constitutes a pioneering approach to engaging marginalised, hard-to-reach and vulnerable populations such as street children, offenders and mental health patients in an intensive, performance-led contemporary dance process. Over the years, this unique methodology has been formalised into a written framework of key features and principles. The positive and often life-changing impact of the work has been previously evaluated through numerous published as well as unpublished research studies (Bramley & Jermyn 2006; Dance United 2014b; Miles & Strauss 2008; Optimity Advisors 2016; van Poortvliet, Joy & Nevill 2010). However, the methodology and its core concepts have never been scholarly examined and embedded in a theoretical framework. I am currently endeavouring to achieve such a theoretical foundation through my PhD research at the Ludwig-Maximilians-University Munich.

I am taking my contribution to this book as an opportunity to assess my personal interdisciplinary perspective on the *Dance United* methodology,

DOI: 10.4324/9781003222484-7

basing it on my own experience of the approach in action as an applied and embodied practice. I contextualise these practice-based insights in relevant theoretical considerations related to my background and expertise as a Dance Movement Psychotherapist.

An interdisciplinary perspective

As an artist, educator and psychotherapist, I bring a unique interdisciplinary perspective to the *Dance United* methodology. In my professional journey before joining the company, I had trained and performed as a professional contemporary dancer, studied pedagogics and also qualified and practised as a Dance Movement Psychotherapist. With this unique professional expertise, I came to the company as a Dance Artist trainee and received extensive on-the-job training over the course of six months. With my therapeutic background, there were initial reservations about me being able to drive the work to the company's high artistic standards, often being reminded that "this is not therapy" despite its therapeutic outcomes for participants. After two years, I had progressed to the role of Dance Director. In this role, I managed the company's *Academy Programme* in London, contributed to the company's choreographic repertoire as well as developed pioneering pilot projects in the mental health sector, which was immensely informed by my insights as a Dance Movement Psychotherapist.

Approaching the work with an interdisciplinary perspective has been both challenging and enriching. Facilitating an artistic performance-led process compared to a process-led therapeutic journey confronted me with a continuous precarious balance between focus on outcome and the individual development of participants. However, understanding the workings of the methodology on a different therapeutic level with informed insights into individual growth and group processes aided me in balancing this tightrope act. Above all, with my interdisciplinary perspective I hold a profound and complex understanding of the common ground the different fields share, that is, the transformative power of dance. I believe therein lies the potential of the transdisciplinary intersection between art, education and therapy.

The work of dance united

> They didn't only teach dance, they gave us life.
> Participant – Adugna Dance Theatre Company (Plastow 2004: 125)

The work of *Dance United* has evolved from the field of British Community Dance, particularly within the context of the social inclusion sector. The beginnings of the organisation however have taken place in the mid-90s in Addis Ababa in Ethiopia, when a collaborative performance project with 120 street and working children brought together Andrew Coggins, a

TV producer, the Ethiopian Gemini Trust, an NGO based in Addis Ababa, and Royston Maldoom, a British dance artist and choreographer (Maldoom 2010). After the successful conclusion of a large-scale performance project, the work further evolved over six years with 18 young Ethiopians and resulted in the formation of the *Adugna Dance Theatre Company* (Plastow 2004). Endeavouring to expand this work and establish it in the UK, Andrew Coggins, Royston Maldoom and Mags Byrne, a choreographer who played an integral role in the work in Ethiopia, founded *Dance United* as a registered UK charity in 2000.

Initially, the work of *Dance United* focused on three international and national key areas, maintaining the core approach of an intensive performance-led contemporary dance process across all activities. These three areas entailed an international strand including projects in Lima, Peru and Germany, community coherence work in the divided socio-political context of Northern Ireland and work in the criminal justice system in England. At this stage of the historical development of *Dance United*, the company felt the need to formalise its practice in order to promote the work and to communicate it externally, acquiring essential funding as well as building networks and partnerships. This constituted the origins of the *Dance United* methodology. The project-based work in prisons gradually evolved into more continuous provisions for young people on parole through the *Academy Programme* in Bradford in 2005 (Miles & Strauss 2008). In 2009, this format was rolled out to Winchester as the *Wessex Dance Academy* and in 2010 the program was set up in London as the *Dance United London Academy*. In 2013, the work successfully expanded into the mental health sector through a project collaboration with the Institute of Psychiatry and the South London and Maudsley NHS foundation trust (Dance United 2014b).

The work of *Dance United* received national as well as international recognition as 'one of the most original and successful youth engagement programs in Britain' (Bennhold 2013: 4). For their outstanding contributions to contemporary dance and marginalised communities, founding members Royston Maldoom and Andrew Coggins were, respectively, awarded an OBE and MBE. The *Academy Programme* received several awards including an Award for Excellence and Innovation in Arts Work with Young People at Risk, the Youth Justice Award and the Koestler Trust Award (Hunter & Gladstone 2009). Despite its proven success rate and track-record, *Dance United* had to close in 2014 due to the adverse outcomes of a cluster of key funding applications. The practical implementation of the *Dance United* methodology continued nonetheless: 'However, all is not lost. Dance United as an approach to contemporary dance will live on…The heart and soul of Dance United survives' (Dance United 2014a). The work thus continued within the context of Dance United Yorkshire and the Destino Dance Company in Ethiopia as well as various project initiatives such as the Alchemy Project in the mental health sector, the Avanti Project with marginalised young people in Kent.

Over the years, the *Dance United* methodology has evolved and was informed by research and evaluations (Bramley & Jermyn 2006; Dance United 2014b; Miles & Strauss 2008; Optimity Advisors 2016; van Poortvliet, Joy & Nevill 2010) as well as by the learning from practical implementation. However, it has always maintained its integrity by adhering to the following core principles. First, all work is performance-led and aims to achieve the highest artistic standards. Second, that the training, rehearsal and performance process is based on professional contemporary dance practice and third that the work is delivered in an intensive and immersive full-time format. The methodology consists of a catalogue of specific pro-active pedagogical strategies guiding the delivery process. Although the strategies are not unique or necessarily novel, in their entirety they describe a specific and pioneering approach of engaging marginalised and vulnerable populations in a process of embodied self-realisation. The company always highlighted that these principles are by no means descriptive, as a successful project delivery is ultimately dependent on the dance artists, their passion and unyielding commitment to their art form and the people with whom they work. The methodological framework serves as a guiding principle for the unique and individual teaching styles of artists in realising the company's core aim 'to advance dance as a tool for personal development and social change' (Dance United 2003: 3).

In my account, I look at two core concepts underlying the principles of the *Dance United* methodology as I consider them crucial and integral mechanisms in facilitating an embodied creative process of personal transformation in the participants. The first methodological concept of offering participants a fresh start in the novel role of a dancer constitutes quite a clash with psychotherapeutic practice. Compared to thorough clinical assessments, it requires the dance artists to actively avoid knowing about participants' histories. In contrast, the second core concept of providing a safe space for learning and growth is a very established principle of therapeutic practice and confirms the importance of structure, containment and boundaries to processes of personal change. Looking at these two different core concepts not only highlights differences and commonalities between therapeutic, educational and artistic practice but it most importantly opens up a dialogue for the enriching potential of interdisciplinary exchange.

Offering a fresh start in the role of a dancer

> You embody the dancer much more than if you were just called a member of the group. So, by being called a dancer, it gives you extra confidence.
> Participant – *Seabreeze*, Mental Health Pilot Project (Dance United 2013)

It is a fundamental principle of the *Dance United* methodology to offer participants a fresh start by welcoming them onto the projects as dancers working towards becoming a dance company: 'We're not interested in anything that you have done in the past; we're not interested in any baggage that you bring with you. When you're here, you're a dancer. And that's all we're interested in' (Dance United 2010).

From very early on in the process, the participants are referred to as 'dancers' collectively working towards a performance as a dance company. The role of a dancer offers a new frame of reference for participants to realise themselves within and to creatively forge a new sense of self. Before joining a project, participants have often held social roles with negative labels such as 'young offender', 'school drop-out', 'gang member', 'deviant' and 'mentally ill'. These stigmatising attributions potentially limit the population *Dance United* worked with in the full realisation of their potentials. The detrimental impact and influence of negative labels and stigma on self-image and social behaviour has been prominently established by labelling theory in the 1960s and 1970s (Macionis & Gerber 2010). Recent research into the effects of labels by example of mental health patients has shown for stigma to be a powerful and persistent influence on their lives resulting in social isolation, negative self-concept as well as low self-esteem and self-worth (Wright, Gronfein & Owens 2000). Especially when working with vulnerable and marginalised populations through dance, it is important to bear in mind that social structures and power relations are not only internalised by way of cognitive self-concepts but also manifest in embodied experiences. Bourdieu's (1977) term habitus, with the body as a bearer of symbolic value, as well as Foucault's (1977) concept of the docile body as a subject to power structures highlight this potential embodiment of social norms and structures of oppression.

By implication, positive labels, such as 'dancer', which is resource-orientated and focuses on individual capabilities, can offer a novel context for exploring new forms of subjectivity and shedding old socially imposed patterns. This is not only a cognitive creative process of re-defining one's self concept but an embodied experience facilitated through the dance. In their research, *Dance United* has termed this outcome 'embodied confidence', firmly locating this process of personal growth in the dance-led process (Miles & Strauss 2008). For example, as one dancer noted: "Even just holding yourself up straight and lifting your head up; like I've started walking with my head up when I walk down the street and I used to walk with it down" (Dance United 2013). In their role as dancers, participants experience themselves and their bodies as capable by mastering movement, gaining strength, exerting control by finding stillness and focus as well as exploring their physical expressivity. In the collective experience of becoming a dance company, they experience themselves as an integral part of a community making valuable contributions and establishing a sense of belonging. On stage, they publicly display themselves as capable and competent, realising their potential and talents. This is often the first time the participants are seen for their achievements by friends, family and carers, the professionals around them as well as the general public, thus powerfully challenging the often negative perceptions about who they are and their capabilities.

This core concept of offering a novel role is particularly effective in relation to the principle of offering participants a 'clean slate'. This methodological principle states that dance artists do not try to find out our participants' backgrounds and actively avoid knowing their history. Working for *Dance United*, I only held information on participants when it was absolutely necessary to facilitating the process safely. This approach was in stark contrast to my practice as a Dance Movement Psychotherapist, which required me to conduct thorough assessments of clients before starting therapy by actively gathering information on their clinical or educational history. This principle of the methodology, thus, initially made me very uncomfortable and raised many question marks around safe containment and adequate support. However, as a thorough assessment and recruitment process by the support team allowed for this information to be present within the multidisciplinary team, the participants were appropriately supported throughout by the team as a whole. It allowed the dance team to focus on the rehearsal process in the dance studio keeping it clear of personal issues and to meet the participants authentically in the moment in their role as dancers. Not only did this methodological principle aid the dance artists in the delivery process, it also helped the participants in shifting their focus away from their issues towards their work in the studio. In the words of one dancer:

> You're not talking about your issues . . . , even though we all have them. You're not on display as it were, so it's not that rawness of it. You're doing something that's fun and everybody is anxious about it . . . so there's a unity in the fact that we're experiencing similar anxieties at those moments and that we are coming together to solve them, to get through it.
>
> (Dance United 2013)

The opportunity of a 'clean slate' combined with the allocation of an unfamiliar and resource-orientated role offers a potential space for participants to discover and re-define their understanding of who they are and to explore creatively who they might want to become. As such, I believe offering a fresh start in the role of a dancer is a fundamental core concept of the *Dance United* methodology, which enables the process of embodied realisation of individual as well as collective potential and catalyses personal transformation.

Offering a safe space to realise potential

> Now when I look back on it, I just think to myself that everything I had never lasts... because I never work hard for it. And that's the most important thing out of the whole project...the fact that someone can focus for that long. If you can focus for that long, you can focus on your dream, your dream of what you want to be.
>
> Participant – *Hidden*, London Academy Pilot Project (Dance United 2010)

Dance United's projects offered a highly focused, structured, immersive and intensive learning environment (Miles & Strauss 2008). Numerous methodological principles underline and frame the importance of providing a contained, protected and tightly planned process for the participants to avoid disengagement and to limit risks. I condense these principles into the core concept of establishing a safe space for personal growth and transformation – "a sanctuary" as a participant once called it.

This core concept is realised throughout all aspects of project planning and delivery. It starts with the choreographic process, which is pre-mapped and ideally trialled before delivering it on a project. The delivery process is planned and tightly structured with gradual stepping stones and a focus on facilitating regular moments of achievement for participants as well as eliminating risks of frustration and disengagement. The client group with which we worked at *Dance United* often led chaotic lives, came with a background of traumatic experiences such as domestic violence, abuse and crime, carried negative self-images and self-limiting beliefs. Our core task was thus to develop a sense of safety and trust as well as a sense of belonging. Having clear boundaries, expectations and objectives helped participants to settle in and engage with their learning. I believe this was fundamental in allowing them to commit and fully engage with a process of self-realisation and personal transformation.

As a Dance Movement Psychotherapist, this core concept of the methodology was evident and most obvious to me. Being familiar with psychotherapeutic principles of establishing a safe space such as Winnicott's *holding* (1960) and Bion's *containment* (1962), I was familiar with the importance of a boundaried space for self-development. Within this core concept however, the idea of a pre-mapped choreography has been a particularly contentious aspect for artists collaborating with *Dance United* but also for other professionals who have come into contact with the work, as they question the creative space this leaves for participants to explore their own personal movement material and ultimately become empowered co-creators in this process. I am not proposing a dogmatic interpretation of the methodological principle of working with a pre-set choreography. I can see the immense benefits a co-creative choreographic process can bring to a project with non-trained dancers from marginalised and vulnerable populations. However, I believe that without the clear choreographic structure and tightly planned delivery, a process of self-development would actually not have been possible to achieve in such a short amount of time in a goal-orientated process.

I best understand the workings of this core concept through Maslow's *Hierarchy of Needs* meeting basic deficiency needs of safety, belonging and esteem first before supporting growth needs of self-actualisation (Maslow 1954). Our first task was, thus, to provide a sense of safety through clear boundaries and consistent structures, including a trust in the rehearsal process. Working together as a dance company towards a performance provided the convivial experience needed to facilitate a sense of belonging in a predictable working process. With regular moments of achievement and a respectful caring working environment, needs of esteem were met. One participant noted poignantly: 'If someone asked me what's successful about the *Academy*, I'd say it's in the way it makes people care. When people go off the rails, there's nothing for them. But when I started going to the Academy, I had a reason to get up in the morning. Something to care about, and people who care about you' (Miles & Strauss 2008: 45).

Within this, the pre-mapped choreography was a vital tool guiding the rehearsal process and meeting needs of safety, belonging and esteem and ultimately working towards self-actualisation. As the choreographic journey was pre-set, we as dance artists could fully focus on delivery and provide a predictable learning journey without extensive moments of creative unknowing and exploring. The choreographic structure provided different roles to accommodate a variety of levels of ability, welcoming and integrating everyone with their individual capacities and strengths. With a wide range of dynamics and qualities as well as different movement material including solos, duets and unison group moments, the choreographies offered a range of different parts. This made the choreographies flexible and accessible for heterogeneous groups of participants, allowing anyone to participate, regardless of shape, size, background, experience or level of fitness. Each participant was challenged within their abilities. It also provided different access points for a variety of learning styles into the learning journey. We carefully placed considerate structured moments of creative exploration with purpose and stages of exploration, always emphasising a sense of achievement to facilitate a sense of pride and confidence. Such explorations were often initially introduced through games to playfully develop basic movement material, which was then further developed through introducing choreographic tools to play with such as spatial directions, levels and orientations, movement dynamics or imagery. Thus, participants experienced their own creative capacities but were not overwhelmed or pressured to produce certain creative outcomes.

With regards to the question of ownership, there always was a clear step towards the end of rehearsals, coming up to the performance, when we as dance artists stepped back and handed the choreography over to the group. They were in charge of being in time for their cues, knowing where they needed to be next. They were in charge of their performance on stage; we were not in the wings but sat in the audience. This was always a deeply empowering moment and although the choreography might not have been developed by them, at that stage of the process, they owned it; they forged their own paths through it and embodied it with their individual meaning as Wilford (2001) explains, 'The notion that the women didn't just do the moves, go through the motions, but actually gave themselves – they owned the moves of the dance, they felt it, they were it, they were convincing and believable' (17).

By providing a safe yet challenging learning environment, the projects met participants in their basic and fundamental needs first before enabling them to attend to and engage with their need for personal development and growth. The methodology's core concept of providing a safe space thus is a vital aspect in facilitating embodied processes of personal transformation.

Critical reflections

In conclusion of my personal interdisciplinary assessment of the core concepts of the *Dance United* methodology, I take the opportunity to highlight an area of concern regarding this work, particularly embedding it in its socio-political context and critically assessing the implications of working with marginalised and vulnerable populations.

My area of concern stems from the issue of instrumentalisation of the arts in the service of socio-politically driven power structures. In this process, art is allocated a function and practised for specific purposes. The intrinsic value of arts practice is lost. The populations *Dance United* worked with were marginalised by society as they were considered deviant from established structures of a neo-liberal capitalist society. It is therefore essential to question if the work of *Dance United* actually contributed to these social power dynamics through turning disengaged members of society into functional and adapted individuals, fitting neatly into norms of productivity. If this is the case, the aim of 'advancing dance as a tool for personal development and social change' (Dance United 2003: 3) actually becomes redundant and a disservice to the populations it endeavours to empower as it reiterates and thus strengthens existing oppressive structures. From my experience of the work, I believe this approach is underpinned by a deep respect for the uniqueness of the art form itself. Such projects can indeed be a means to an end, but the intrinsic potential can only be fully realised by dancing for dancing's sake.

When evaluating the work and proving its efficacy to potential funders and partners, the company focused on established indicators of social codes and norms such as offending rates, engagement with education and employment as well as acquisition of transferrable skills and competencies. An analysis of the socio-economic impact of the work even highlighted the cost effectiveness and viability of investment at a 215% return (van Poortvliet, Joy & Nevill 2010). However, the research on the outcomes always struggled to capture and describe the impact of the work comprehensively by means of standardised and established evaluation frameworks. The work of *Dance United* operated in the often-conflicting interplay between economic needs for funding the work and its artistic and social aspiration to enable and engage marginalised populations in their empowerment and realisation of potential. Within this context it becomes very telling that ultimately the company had to close due to financial difficulties.

How do you put a number on the 'young offender', who arrived on the project with an extremely short attention span and such low frustration tolerance level that he kicked-off almost every day, reminding me to tell everyone to stay focused before the performance and fighting his way through a

20-minute choreography with concentration and commitment throughout, without any wings behind which to hide. Or the 'mental health patient', who could not look anyone in the eye or hold a conversation, standing confidently in the spotlight with her head held high dancing the opening solo at a packed theatre in central London.

There are countless such moments of profound transformation I have witnessed, which deeply move and touch me to this day. I am still humbled by the courage of the people I was lucky enough to work with, who trusted me to accompany them on a journey to discover their potential and own their worth. Having been witness to these journeys, I can attest that the work of *Dance United* has indeed empowered participants in ways beyond socially prescribed categories such as transferrable skills and competencies. It reminded them of what they are capable of: their innate human capacity to shape and forge their own unique path through life.

Therein lies the transformative potential of dance shared across the disciplines of therapy, education and art.

References

Annable-Coop, C. (2016). A powerful catalyst. *Animated – the Community Dance Magazine*, Spring, pp. 14–16.

Bennhold, K. (2013). Giving youth a chance to leap and soar. *New York Times*, August 14th (4) Retrieved from https://www.nytimes.com/2013/08/15/world/europe/giving-troubled-youth-a-chance-to-turn-it-around.html.

Bion, W. (1962). *Learning From Experience*. London: Karnac Books.

Bourdieu, P. (1977). *Outline of a Theory of Practice*. Cambridge: Cambridge University Press.

Bramley, I., & Jermyn, H. (2006). *Dance Included - Towards Good Practice in Dance and Social Inclusion*. Marston Book Services.

Dance United. (2003). *Directors' and Trustees' Report and Financial Statement*. Companies House.

Dance United. (2010). Hidden. Moonmanmedia / Duet Pictures Production. Unpublished promotional video.

Dance United. (2013). Seabreeze – A Four-Week Pilot Project in Mental Health. Unpublished promotional video.

Dance United. (2014a). An Important Message by our Chair of Trustees. Retrieved from https://web.archive.org/web/20141003184507/http://www.dance-united.com/article/important-message-our-chair-trustees.

Dance United. (2014b). Seabreeze: South London Mental Health Pilot Project Evaluation Report. Unpublished evaluation report.

Foucault, M. (1977). *Discipline and Punish: The Birth of the Prison*. London: Penguin Books.

Hunter, V., & Gladstone, P. (2009). Dance and social inclusion: Facilitating the process, developing graduate employability. *The International Journal of the Arts in Society*, 4(2), pp. 149–159.

Macionis, J., & Gerber, L. (2010). *Sociology* (7th ed.). London: Pearson Education Canada.

Maldoom, R. (2010). Tanz um dein Leben: meine Arbeit, meine Geschichte. Fischer Verlag.

Maslow, A.H. (1954). *Motivation and Personality*. New York: Harper & Row.

Miles, A., & Strauss, P. (2008). The Academy - A Report on Outcomes for Participants. ESRC Centre for Research on Socio-cultural Change, University of Manchester.

Optimity Advisors. (2016). The Alchemy Project Evaluation Report. Retrieved from https://www.artshealthresources.org.uk/docs/the-alchemy-project-evaluation-report/.

Plastow, J. (2004). Dance and transformation: The Adugna dance theatre, Ethiopia. In Boon, R. & Plastow, J. (eds.), *Theatre and empowerment: Community drama and the world stage*, pp. 125–154. Cambridge: Cambridge University Press.

van Poortvliet, M., Joy, I., & Nevill, C. (2010). Trial and Error: Children and Young People in Trouble with the Law. New Philanthropy Capital.

Wilford, S. (2001). Dance United HMP Holloway Project - Evaluation and Impact Assessment. Unpublished evaluation report.

Winnicott, D. (1960). The theory of the parent-child relationship. *International Journal of Psychoanalysis*, 41, pp. 585–595.

Wright, E.R., Gronfein, W.P., & Owens, T.J. (2000). Deinstitutionalization, social rejection, and the self-esteem of former mental patients. *Journal of Health and Social Behavior*, 41(1), pp. 68–90.

8 Breath, belly and back. Dropping into body as ground

Paul Beaumont

Introduction

Heart beating
Breath, cold stinging air in my nostrils
Dry mouth, moistening, tasting
Shifting to feel my feet
Breathing deeply – cool air in nostrils
Teeth jaw tight, yawn to release

Belly soft
Shifting weight
Bony back, flexing spinal sequence

Generating heat
Making NOISE, receiving quiet.

Changing direction, coming to the floor,
Widening arms, breathing deeply
Opening, closing

Seeing what I see, registering the room, the trees, the quiet

Connecting with my visceral body, internal space and substance. Bone and gristle, full and empty, soft tissue organs, emotional waters, pleasant or un-eased?

Breathing to settle

Registering ground, allowing head to rise, my vertical human to be ready. Ready in stillness, ready to move, ready to meet. Holding space, inside and outside. Breathing back and ground.

DOI: 10.4324/9781003222484-8

This is an account of what I track in myself on arrival in the studio, preparing to meet someone I'm working with. It is this connection with the resource of the alive body, that holds my creative potential, that I bring to this chapter. I see the practice of 're-sourcing' as being one where I return repeatedly to a source, a start, a beginning and a ground. And I see this source as being the felt experience of the body and movement.

I am advocating the value of dropping down into the body, where I can sense, notice and track my moving and breathing experience. I want to support the wider trusting of this practice and the value of giving it space. As I return to the body, finding expression both non-verbal and verbal, I value the unfolding process.

In the first part of this chapter, I offer the context in which I reclaim this felt experience, naming its privilege and how external pressures and avoidance can have an impact. I name the part that the supportive approaches of Body Mind Centering® and Authentic Movement have played, together with some of the developmental origins that hold the foundation of attending to my felt sense.

In the second part, I describe the process when working with another, using brief fictionalised accounts of the stages my work with a client might pass through. I name the preliminary stages of noticing, orientation, safety, space and boundary. I then visit the stages of creative expression of working with what is present, embodied wisdom and body intelligence, and an ability to hold the unknown. I close with an acknowledgement of what is harvested and reflected upon.

Interspersed through the chapter are explorations that are designed to support your connection with your own body. They illustrate elements of my practice that I want to share and are for you to try, as stepping stones as you read. So please have a break from reading and take time to pause and follow the exploration.

I write from my standpoint as a Somatic Movement practitioner. Somatic Movement is an umbrella term to describe a number of practices that acknowledge the value of working with the 'felt sense' – our subjective experience of being human that is grounded in the body (Gendlin 2003; Hannah 1988).

I offer here my view on the significance of returning to the body, movement and our felt sense, as a home base to return to, again and again. I present the value of this in itself, for insight, release, liberation and healing and a way to cultivate acceptance, compassion, connection and wisdom.

EXPLORATION: ARRIVAL.

How is your body right now?
Where are you in contact with the ground?
What's the shape of your breath?
As you notice, what settles or changes?

A somatic movement practice – returning to the body

The nature of practice

When I practise something, I return to it again and again. I 'put' something 'in' to practice, so it's about applying something, a conscious choice, rather than just a theory about it. My practice can be a ritual that can respect and honour its significance and contribution. I value this commitment to return to the body and movement with a beginner's mind. I am advocating this as a resource for all, for the practitioner and a foundation in working with others.

I also want to highlight the phenomenon of 'dropping down' as I move. I breathe out, exhaling and releasing weight, so I can feel the support of the earth beneath me. At the bottom of the outbreath, there is a pause, a quiet moment to notice what I am with, before the inhale comes, where there is a filling, a rising extension of my spine, supported by a push into the ground. This is an expression of my autonomic nervous system that manages the involuntary, unconsciously controlled, internal functions of the body. The outbreath is linked with the parasympathetic state of the autonomic nervous system, and the inbreath shifts into the sympathetic state. The nervous system can support this flow between inward and outward sensing; alert expression serves as a contribution to our embodied, creative process.

The dropping down can also be representative of shifting the focus of the attention of my nervous system. I might initially need to close my eyes, reducing the input to the visual system, enabling me to give greater attention to other interoception senses. I can begin to feel more viscerally when I am not receiving information from the outer world visually. Over time, I can move more easily between the two, choosing between an inner and outer focus.

Reclaiming the felt experience

In my experience, the wider culture I have lived in (white dominant and patriarchal) tends not to value the somatic, the felt experience, the phenomenon of what it is to experience ourselves through our own unique perception. And yet my experience of this culture, with its level of privilege, offers conditions of enough safety, with basic needs met, to enable me to turn inwards and attend to my felt sense.

No doubt in earlier times, and still in many places in the world, the focus is on survival, on carrying on, on keeping busy out of necessity of the task at hand. I am reminded of the response my elderly mother often offers, when I tell her about my week: 'Well, as long as you're keeping busy'. Perhaps this reflects a certain generational perspective that came out of a war-time coping strategy: Keeping busy so as not to feel what is painful or difficult. Perhaps it reflects a certain production-based work ethic. I get caught in answering emails rather than attending to what I actually want to focus on.

EXPLORATION – FILLING THE FRAME, FOLLOWING SENSATION:

This practice can hold the creative track – as you focus on where you are, the next step emerges and your path unfolds.

- Imagine as you move or sit, you are in a film.
- Fill out the 'frame' of your current position. Name to yourself what you notice, through sensation? 'I feel my heels on the floor, the air in my nose, a heaviness and pressure at the back of my skull'.
- Allow the 'frame by frame' of your body experience to be as full as it is, and flow into change. Notice how the next frame arises, without you having to consciously do anything. Your job is simply to fill your present moment frame by noticing what you sense.
- Follow the physical tone of your body. 'My head falls forward and my neck lengthens'.
- Follow the emotional tone of your body. 'I feel a quiet peacefulness … and a dullness arises too as I curl forward'.

Supportive approaches

During my life I have found particular movement forms and approaches to have been profoundly influential and provided foundational stepping stones for me as a practitioner. These include Contact Improvisation, Body Mind Centering® (BMC) and Authentic Movement.

Contact Improvisation offered a practice where there were no steps to learn or shapes to get my body to make. Here, an improvised, relational and sensory dialogue created the flow of the movement. Following on from this, the experiential nature of Bonnie Bainbridge Cohen's BMC® work contributed enormously to my practice of following my felt-sense:

> [T]he challenge is to not be confined by what we have already learned but to continually allow our discoveries to pass into our unconscious and to approach each moment with trust and innocence.
>
> (Bainbridge Cohen 1993: 2)

BMC's approach explores anatomy and physiology of the body through ki-naesthetic and proprioceptive experience. How I move and how I sense that movement helps me notice my visceral, bodily experience. As I begin to notice and differentiate my experience of my lungs for example, from the sensation in my belly, I can begin to name, value and relate to each aspect more deeply. My moment by moment lived experience has a place that I can ground in the stuff of my body.

In addition, the practice of Authentic Movement (Adler 2002) has supported an ability to arrive in an empty space, as I close my eyes and listen inwardly to arising impulses as they change. I track the layers of experience of body, sensation, feeling and image and can use this framework to support personal practice and work with others. Where am I, where are they in these four layers? I find ways to separate out and articulate my experience.

EXPLORATION: A BRIEF CHECK IN FOR YOUR BODY.

Bring your awareness to your physical body.
How is your back?
How is your front?
Allow them to move and adjust for more comfort.
What do they have to say right now?

The ground of the body

The practices described above have enriched my felt-sense from the inside out. They support a foundation that my body offers, a ground that I can land on and push off from, into expression, creativity and change. These are practices that come from my sensing body rather than an external expert or aesthetic. They offer a deep and grounded respect for the body. Whatever I might be feeling, I can always return to what I sense and move from there. I can exercise and hone the ability to pay attention to myself without judgement and practise this when working with others therapeutically. For the more I can feel myself, the more I can feel of others (Siegel 2018). This builds connection, internal and external.

I sense the body, to notice and feel the information my sensory nervous system is picking up, moment by moment. I might feel tone or pressure. I might notice the overlapping of physical sensation with an experience of a particular feeling quality. This may have a rising or growing quality or falling and fading one, as the 'volume' of what I experience shifts and changes. I might name an experience in my body and give it the title 'anxiety' or 'excitement'. As I do so, I can gradually begin to separate out the emotion and sensation. This enables me to find a new place to stand and a potentially new starting point to explore from.

Developmental foundations – the beginnings of creativity

I'm in my local Children's Centre running a movement play session for babies and dads/male carers. A dad arrives with a sleeping newborn, curled into his chest and cradled by his arms. I can see the contrast with the six-month-old baby, on the ground, lifting their head and finding the push from their arms, face alert.

I can witness this transition, from the 'yes' of bonding with a parent to the beginnings of separating and finding the assertive 'no' through the push of our arms:

[T]he child begins the transition from a state of being merged with another to one of greater independence and autonomy as an individual
(Hartley 1989: 70).

This is the early expression of will, volition and choice. A basic expression of an impulse and direction that underlies all creative acts. And between the push of the no and reach towards the yes, there is a transitional place, a creative space of potential and transformation. For many of us, the creative space is opened up in sensory play.

It is in the infant's actual experience of making the transitions that they learn, grow and develop their sense of individuality and competence in the world: 'Within this play we create a space in which the transition of transformation may take place' (Hartley 1994: 106).

Early in infant development, a baby might spontaneously engage with the changing light landing on their face as they move an arm. They might play with the feeling of a blanket on their toes. They are unconsciously called to engage in this meaningful sensory exploration. The early, pre-verbal months inhabit this realm of body, sensation, emotion and movement as spontaneity becomes exploration and experimentation. Stern (1990) reflects on the experience of a six-week-old infant: 'Imagine that none of the things you see or touch or hear have names or functions, and few any memories attached to them' (13). He describes how we respond towards or away from different levels of intensity of sensory experience – touch, sound, light etc. Entering into this sensory, emotional realm, our play and creativity begins. All this happens without word or higher cognitive understanding, and somatic practices support this 'dropping down' into foundational, sensory experiences.

I am advocating the value of hanging out here. Of not rushing on too quickly to find cognitive meaning, but to truly prize the phase of creativity where we 'don't know', but maybe splash about a bit in the waters of where we find ourselves. Back at the Children's Centre we are all on the floor, hanging out together:

I mirror how the babies are – lying on backs, playing with feet; Swaying legs in the air, or reaching and turning the head, to come into a roll. A crawler makes their way across the room, Dad follows, and a stop-start game emerges. Adults try things out, and with encouragement words fall away.

There is something particular about non-verbal play. An offering, a dialogue and an exchange can emerge, when I 'drop down' into the felt sense, as something both individual and shared is explored. It does not need to be named, and yet I know something is going on that is meaningful – there is a connection alongside the creative exploration.

EXPLORATION: A PERSONAL PROCESS OF EMBODIED CREATIVITY.

Consider the following stages to support your own non-verbal, embodied beginnings of creativity.

1   *Pre-conditions.* What is needed for you to feel safe, held or relaxed enough to return to your body? What do you need to set up practically?
2   *Warming up phase.* Arrival. What is needed here? Movement, the ordinary stretch, the run or dance? Connect with breath, skin, bones and muscles.
3   *Take some space, Make some noise* to be with what you receive through your senses. Follow your energy or focus. Allow a movement, gesture, shape or line of travel. What needs to be stirred up or allowed to come into form? What needs to be offered to the space, or received? Is there an encounter that needs to happen in the space?
4   *Being with the unknown.* Letting your body lead the way. Your mind can stand back.
5   *Returning to ground.* Resting, receiving gravity. Noticing what is present.
6   *Mark making* as an extension or expression of movement. Let the drawing draw itself, without judgement.
7   *Optional:* finding words, writing, sharing, reflecting and harvesting to take forward.

Meeting others

At the beginning of the chapter, I described the ritual of arriving ready to work with another. Checking practicalities in the room and props needed contributes to the conditions of safety. Then noticing what I am with in my body, I can let go into a small flow of movement-sensory experience. I inhabit the substance of my body, shifting from belly to muscles and bones. I contact the ground as a counterpoint to emotional energy. I connect with joints to support flexibility and responsiveness. So, in preparation to meet with another, the process of embodied creativity is drawn upon. I find safety, tune into senses and bring this into expression.

I can draw on this practice too after a session, to notice what I might have received and what lingers for me following work with someone. I can use this to reflect on the meaning of the work and the terrain we are in. I can also use the practice to move through what I might have been left with, to bring it into expression, release it into the space, and reconnect with myself.

The process of reclaiming embodied creativity

As a somatic practitioner, I see the creative process as one that encompasses being with what is known or unknown, attending to what arises, moment by moment, through the body – its movement, sensations, feelings, images and associations. I hold the space for the expression of that and see what emerges. Somatic creativity is the process of change and realisation that comes from sensing and expressing.

In this second part of the chapter, I will describe a number of stages this process moves through, that come from my personal movement practice, and how this applies to my work with clients. I see the process as follows and highlight the stages working with an adult client:

1   Those I work with might initially notice a dissatisfaction or desire and seek something for themselves;
2   They orientate and find safety, as they continue to sense;
3   Something is brought into expression;
4   Our discoveries can then be harvested and cherished.

Noticing and seeking

> For some time, my client has not been feeling well, some low-grade back pain, a series of colds and general low energy for life, both physical and emotional. Their work has not been satisfying and motivation can be hard to find.

This is an example of how a client may be at an early stage of registering that something is out of kilter and not as it might be. A discomfort is present or a feeling of the absence or loss of something. Equally a major life incident may mean that they are forced to stop, to pay attention. They have no choice – their regular strategies and patterns may not be effective. They might then have the impulse to reach out, to seek something, to know more. The first impulse is to move in a new direction and enquire into what else might be possible.

EXPLORATION: A BRIEF CHECK IN FOR YOUR BODY.

How is your belly and centre?
How is your head and tail?
Shift your feet or turn your head.
What brings a feeling of freedom or space inside?

Orientating and finding safety

A principle drawn from BMC® is that of support preceding movement. Stability before mobility. We can see this in functional movement – a stable base or core enables flexible movement around that point. In infant movement development, the baby establishes contact with the ground first, as it yields and bonds, before it pushes away or reaches out (Hartley 1995). Psychologically too, we need safety before we can explore. It is why our attachment figures are so important (Bowlby 1988). It is why I close the door before I start work with a group. It is why I speak to clients about the optional use of touch in my work, so that they can give informed consent each time this is offered. Feeling safe enough is a pre-requisite for the creative process:

> After reading information on my website, my client made initial contact via an email, followed by a phone call, and we have decided to meet in the studio for an initial session of how it might be to work together.

So here, my client is establishing their sense of safety. Finding out information to understand what might be possible, gaining some sense of the territory. They need to feel safe enough, welcome and received, to find their ground and take a few breaths, before they shift their weight off-centre and step in:

> At any kind of transition point in our lives we all need the certainty of knowing at some level that we are securely held. This is the ground from which we leap, however near or far, and to which we can return and be welcomed back.
>
> (Hartley 1994: 109)

Clear space and boundary

Many therapeutic practices have at their foundation the idea of holding a contained space. This can be manifest in the physical environment worked in, the time boundaries in place, together with the background practical and administrative tasks of a professional role that enables work to happen. For the client to come 'home' to their body and their creative, healing process to begin, they need to have a sense of there being a respected and protected space for them. How sessions are facilitated is also significant, with the continuum between freedom and structure. With too much freedom a client might feel lost, with too much structure, they might feel restricted. This is an active process, orientated around what is manageable for the client.

Beginning with the familiar

> After a few minutes of talking in this initial session, I invite my client to come to their feet and have a walk around the space. Welcoming them to

look at the room, taking in this new environment, what is familiar, what is new. Exploration continues with guiding them to notice contact with the floor; the phrase of the in and out breath; and noticing the experience of the front body and the back body. They offer a few words to describe tiredness and stiff pain. I invite them to let their ordinary body find the way to be as comfortable as they can and they come to the floor. We bring in blankets and a cushion, and talk some more about what they notice.

After a while, they take the offer of some hands-on work, choosing where contact would feel right. I rest my hand on their back, giving time to receive the contact, not doing or striving. A deep breath rises and falls, their body softens, and the work begins.

So, we start with something of the ordinary – a walk. Noticing what we notice, giving some breathing space. I am not trying to 'do' or change, but take some time to pay attention. I am aiming to build a sense of safety, through holding the space, offering permission and supporting my client to feel some of the substance of their body and self. Beginning this process of reclaiming, I am initially not driving forward for change, but finding resources and comfort, before moving into wider exploration. I begin with what is known and possible: '[We] work first with what is easy and comfortable [. . .] we play between giving support to whatever is happening and holding the vision of what is possible' (Hartley 1994: 106).

Coming into expression

What is present?

In working with others, as well as my own movement practice, I hold a commitment to attending to what is present as best I can. For self or other there might be uncomfortable states, confused places or low energy, as well as clarity, aliveness and direction. It is important to be able to be with the full spectrum of experience. Can I welcome the mundane as well as the intense?

Creatively, it can be invaluable to keep open to all the resources available, the spontaneous as well as the planned. Noticing the wider field of what arises, what I might initially see as disturbances or distractions can sometimes have a contribution to make in the creative process. This might be picking up on the energy of the fly that will not settle in the room, my response to the sound of the emergency siren passing by, or the physical resources of the stack of chairs from the corridor being brought in to change the environment to work in. All these resources can contribute to the unfolding creative process.

Embodied wisdom

Physical, emotional or relational patterns and symptoms can keep presenting themselves. Somatic approaches give opportunities to listen and pay attention to other stories and meanings that the symptom or behaviour may hold:

At a later session, my adult client speaks about symptoms of on-going stress and anxiety. I suggest they come into the space to arrive and move to see what their body might have to say. After a short period of movement they describe a wider professional choice about the direction of their work that they are grappling with. As they speak their fingers and hands are actively engaged, and as they amplify this, the movement comes into their whole body and fills the space. They catch their breath and begin to describe what holding this dilemma has been like. Emotional material comes through.

EXPLORATION:

As you sit, is your energy rising or falling?

Is there a subtle pull towards rest or desire to get moving?

Follow your impulse to adjust in response. Make this visible, even for a moment or in a small way.

Body intelligence

Embodied creativity draws on the wealth of our Body Intelligence – what our body knows intuitively, without word or concept (Claxton 2015). This is developed in the infant's early months; they grapple with it through childhood and it can often get lost in adult years. Body intelligence gives someone direction, in the movement towards or away from something. The grumblings in our belly, the tightness in a muscle, the spontaneous flick of a hand as our head turns away – all indicate a knowing or a story to be told that is part of our creative process.

Over time, an understanding of what the body 'knows', beyond words, has grown academically and informs practice in many fields of health and therapy. As neuroscience has developed, and the crossover between this and psychotherapeutic work has evolved, more credence is being paid to this area of human experience. There is now more understanding and acceptance of these unconscious aspects of the nervous system as being key and holding something for personal recovery (Dana 2018; Rothschild 2000; van der Kolk 2014).

In holding the focus on listening to the body, my aim as a practitioner is to witness and support the liberation of my client's personal truth. This can then contribute to the integration of earlier embodied experiences into a wider personal life-story at a pace that is manageable. Once expressed, it can hold less power and influence so that other choices of how to be and relate can come through. Or, it can more consciously, rather than unconsciously be brought forward to drive a person's direction in life.

Holding the 'not knowing'

The holding of the physical, therapeutic space enables the state of being seen without judgement and a creative process to emerge and be told. At times I have to stand back, to simply go with the process, and trust the themes that are returned to again and again. I observe, I support, I take part, I run with the flow. Sometimes, I consciously know what is being worked through; at other times, I am less sure, other than it being meaningful to the client. Conscious meaning can arise more slowly, as pieces are put together, and reflective practice and supervision offer new perspectives. Sometimes, the work is held by the story, the imaginative theme, that creates the safety for the creative space, to enable the sensory and relational work to happen. Returning to my client:

> They share their unease and agitation. The movement has settled, but they are left staring at their two up-turned palms, as if weighing something up. Again, after sharing a little about the two choices, I invite them to take some time to move each one in the movement space.

In offering a space to move in, I am facilitating the small but profound, political and personal act of holding space for the body. In the wider culture of medicine, healthcare and the associated complementary fields of therapy, when consulting with the professional, the expert, we place ourselves in their hands. We bring something that we do not know what to do with, and hope that they will. In this act of giving over to another, the culture can build a pressure that the other 'will know what to do'. So, a tension around expectation can emerge in the professional, as a 'treatment' is expected, a thing to do, as the client hopes to be told 'if you do A, then B will happen'.

A somatic approach holds a pause, a space where other possibilities might emerge. In this act, I am reclaiming a space for the body's creative processes to come through. Creativity can arise when we step back from words and return to the body, to bring into balance both the conscious and unconscious. In facilitating others, I am holding the space for each and aim to enable transition between the two.

Cherishing what was found. Returning, re-gathering, harvesting

> Having moved the two choices in the space my client shares a realisation. "Well of course, I know straight away which one I want, which one I have an alive connection with. That feels so strong." They go on to describe how elements of what was important to them in their work and life have got side-tracked. We reflect together on what got lost, what needs nurturing and given more space as they move forward. My client does a final piece of movement to anchor this in their body.

So, as a client steps into the space, material arises when they can both let go and pay attention. They let go of needing to know, name or understand, and feel into sensation and movement and they let their body speak. Coming to the end of the arc of our exploration, as my client pauses, they can reflect. When ready they can find their words to name their experience and integrate it from bodily to conscious understanding. What can then follow and build is an assertive, powerful and active bringing of something back, a return of the pendulum. There then can be a taking care of, a holding, a cherishing what is now brought close. If needed, any grief of what was lost, or joy and celebration of what has been found can be expressed. With time, what is reclaimed can be integrated, built upon and form a new ground of what they know.

Conclusion

As a practitioner, I believe that my creativity is reclaimed through an ongoing commitment for connection with the moving body. This involves an ability to drop down into the body's flow of movement and sensation, in its evolving process. This holds a willingness to follow the edge of tracking what is known, moment by moment, and how it meets the edge of what is not known. As a Somatic Movement Therapist, I value going slowly, breathing, feeling my ground and applying myself to be attuned to the condition of those I work with. I support those I work with to re-source with the body through the grounded exploration of the moving body:

> I take an outbreath
> My gaze lowers,
> I do a small jiggle and sway, as if shaking something, like sifting soil, to see what is left behind.
> I deepen my contact with the ground,
> I feel and know where I am
> I then push, feel my strength, power,
> I feel my self.
> My spine lengthens, my head rises, my eyes open, I see the world and the world can see me.

References

Adler, J. (2002). *Offering from the conscious body.* Rochester, Vermont: Inner Traditions.

Bainbridge Cohen, B. (1993). *Sensing, feeling and action – The experiential anatomy of body-mind centering.* Northampton, MA, USA: Contact Editions.

Bowlby, J. (1988). *A secure base: Parent-child attachment and healthy human development.* New York: Basic Books.

Chodorow, J. (1991). *Dance therapy and depth psychology – The moving imagination.* London: Routledge.

Claxton, G. L. (2015). *Intelligence in the flesh: Why your mind needs your body much more than it thinks.* New Haven & London: Yale University Press.

Dana, D. (2018). *The polyvagal theory in therapy – Engaging the rhythm of regulation*. New York/London: W.W. Norton.

Gendlin, E. (2003). *Focusing*. London: Rider - Random House.

Hannah, T. (1988). *Somatics: Reawakening the mind's control of movement, flexibility & health*. USA: De Capo.

Hartley, L. (1994). *Wisdom of the body moving – An introduction to body mind centering*. California: North Atlantic Books.

Rothschild, B. (2000). *The body remembers – The psychophysiology of trauma and trauma treatment*. New York & London: W.W. Norton.

Siegel, D. (2018). *Aware: The science and practice of presence*. London: Scribe.

Stern, D. (1990). *Diary of a baby – What your child sees, feels and experiences*. New York: Basic Books.

van der Kolk, B. (2014). *The body keeps the score – Mind, brain and body in the transformation of trauma*. New York: Penguin.

9 'Is that yoga or are you just making it up?'

Helen Poynor

As I was practising movement on Bondi beach in Sydney, a curious passer-by asked, 'Is that yoga or are you just making it up?'. The answer is, of course, that as practitioners, therapists, artists and human beings we are always to some extent 'just making it up' whatever our background, training and experience (and particularly in the light of an accumulated body of experience). Because we are working in the present, in the presence of living beings, moving bodies and feelings, in a live creative process, our response, however considered and theoretically informed, needs to incorporate our own aliveness and a degree of spontaneity if we are to genuinely connect with the experience of the person or group before us. Just as there is not a comprehensive, one size fits all map to show us how to lead our lives, although our values/ethics, upbringing, social and cultural environment and spiritual and political beliefs inform our choices, in each moment of our creative and therapeutic practice there are a multiplicity of possible responses. Although we may pause to draw breath, to 'check' our own condition (emotionally, mentally and physically) or to ask for guidance,[1] even the decision to wait, to say or do nothing, is a choice. I would suggest that our choices frequently arise intuitively from the depths of ourselves beyond conscious thought. It is in the response to our response, that we may begin to understand why or how we have touched our client's or student's reality and how to proceed. The process then repeats itself in a continual unfolding. Engaging with other human beings as a dance movement therapist is necessarily a creative endeavour, a process of improvisation. Any performer who improvises will confirm that improvisation is a finely tuned skill, especially when playing with others. That moment in time with the other person in their (and our) current condition or weather will never recur. Our response to it will alter the next moment and so on in a sequence which could be compared to gradually unfolding a map, or turning the pages of a narrative, or wiping the sand away from a buried drawing. Although it is crucial that our conscious processes are engaged in our work with others, I would argue that they are frequently neither fast enough, nor finely tuned enough nor far reaching enough to adequately respond to the unfolding process in the room, unless they are supported by other levels of knowing. In fact, I suspect that our conscious choices are generally underpinned by the

DOI: 10.4324/9781003222484-9

knowledge and information we are receiving in other ways, including kin-aesthetically and intuitively.

I am aware of the potential pitfalls and dangers of such an approach. A developed level of consciousness is a pre-requisite for any practising therapist, combined with in-depth training and ongoing supervision, but our approach as dance movement therapists needs to be wholistic, incorporating not only the whole person before us, and a spectrum of approaches and ways of moving, but also the whole of us as therapists and fellow human beings.

What can the body reveal to us that language can't? This is the territory of our work.

In my own therapeutic and artistic journey, I have frequently had the experience of being able to express and explore personal issues through movement and autobiographical performance practice before (often years before) I have been able to articulate them through language or work with them consciously in a therapeutic context.

Kinaesthetic exploration does not always have to be mediated by or translated into language in order for it to be therapeutically effective. Sometimes it will go deeper and reveal more, precisely because it is experienced directly through the body and expressed through an embodied creative process rather than corralled by language and rational thought. Some issues and eras in our history are literally too hot to handle if engaged with directly just as looking at the sun can damage our eyes. There are things we may be unable to think or talk about which our moving body and creative imagination may allow us to engage with and process nonetheless. Allowing our work to be circumscribed by our conscious thought processes may prevent us, both as therapists and as clients, from garnering the benefits of other ways of knowing, understanding and integrating our experiences.

Moving itself is a way of the body and the being thinking and reflecting, as well as sensing, feeling and expressing. Processes that we need to follow and attend to, rather than attempt to control or shape, in order to be able to discern the narrative or pattern that is being revealed. At the same time, there may be a level of awareness and a continual process of choice operating as we move, a state of embodied awareness, of the body in the mind and the mind in the body.

We may subsequently choose to engage in a further process of reflection through language, which, although helpful in some cases, is not necessarily essential and could at times simply muddy the waters obscuring or diluting something that is already complete in itself.

Many years ago, I worked for some time with a client[2] who after a brief discussion of her life circumstances and the issues she wished to address said little in our sessions but simply chose to move. She always moved with her back to me at some distance away. It felt important that I respected her choices and what appeared to be a need for privacy in a held and witnessed space where she had permission to move in whatever way felt right for her. Any intervention from me would, I felt, be intrusive and inappropriate. After some time she felt that the process was complete. These sessions required a level of humility from me, an acceptance of not knowing and trust in her innate bodily wisdom. It was her process not mine.

There is a level at which both the therapeutic and the creative process remain 'beyond our ken'; however much we study and practise them, they remain and perhaps must remain shrouded in mystery. Who are we to steal fire from the gods?

Reducing the human condition to the confines of logic and rational thought might foster the illusion that we are in control but denies us the possibility of embracing the whole story. As the mystic Rumi reminds us:

> The inner working of a human being
> is a jungle.

> (Barks 2006: 187)

We are beginning to recognise the price we are paying for attempting to tame the wilderness.

There is a place for language as part of the practice of movement when words arise directly from it, issuing forth from the moving body in embodied language rather than describing, analysing or commenting on it. The issue is not to prioritise the words at the expense of the movement. When I am working in this way myself, I find it necessary to use a delicate process of discernment so that the words do not run away with themselves taking over the show while my movement becomes less and less embodied.

Some years ago, unable to travel to Sydney to an old friend's funeral, my partner and I attended the ceremony on zoom. This enabled us to be present with the other members of our community in the commemoration of her life for which we were grateful, but it was a profoundly disorientating experience, sitting at the computer in pyjamas in the early hours of the morning as the sun rose behind us.

Some hours later, I was fortunate enough to have a continuing professional development exchange with Caroline Frizell with whom I have an ongoing peer relationship (see Chapter 17: The matriarch and the mollusc and all things in between pp. 180–189). I had warned her that I may be in a somewhat altered state as a result of both lack of sleep and the powerful emotions likely to have been evoked. I had not anticipated quite how dissociated I would feel. With Caroline witnessing, I started ricocheting around the room trusting the relationship enough not to censure whatever impulses arose. I felt crazy with no sense of how what I was doing connected to the experience I had just had. In fact, nothing made sense and I didn't care. Messing around rather manically I started playing with a beautiful long-haired toy white rabbit I had spotted, chattering inconsequentially to it while lying on the floor. Behaving for all intents and purposes like an out of control child. This continued for some time. Gradually without either conscious focus or intention, this process enabled me to re-connect with my body and with my feelings.

My emotional and physical state shifted. As I landed in myself, a door opened generating a sequence of movement and words that conjured the atmosphere and experience of the funeral into the small studio in Devon. This gave form to and communicated my experience and feelings, summoning the individuals and community participating in the funeral into the room.

Sometime later I realised the significance of the rabbit, both my friend and her partner were born in the Chinese year of the rabbit which we had often joked about.

Attending the funeral on zoom (my first experience of the platform) was essentially a disembodied experience and only by re-grounding it in my body could I begin to process it. But the bridge back to my kinaesthetic body and my feelings was not immediately accessible to me. I believe that simply making a decision to move from my experience of the funeral would not have resulted in such a fully embodied expression, I needed to traverse my internal chaos first in order to be able to access this. Equally talking about the experience (which would have felt, I suspect, both inaccessible and pointless in the state I was in) would not have reached the same depth or allowed me to integrate it so fully.

I am making an impassioned plea for the primacy of the moving body, at the heart of our practice as dance movement therapists. Coupled with a deeper recognition of the value of the therapist's embodied presence, the importance of not knowing, of humility, spontaneity, creativity and intuition in our work with others. Foregrounding movement itself, not only as a means of exploration and expression, but as a therapeutic medium, a process of resolving and integrating challenging emotions, personal issues and dilemmas, and psychological tensions. Valuing kinaesthetic intuition and embodied language as alternative ways of knowing and understanding our life experiences. Learning to trust enough to follow what arises in an untrammelled way, to not always know what we are doing, to be prepared to stand under something rather than to reduce it to something we understand.[3]

Movement offers a means to drop more deeply into ourself, an invitation to breathe, to land, to re-member who we are, creating space among the busyness of daily life, non-stop activity and continuous mental 'chatter' to listen and reflect from a deeper layer of being. Embodied movement provides an antidote to the increasing cultural pressure towards virtually mediated relationships accompanied by a corresponding distrust of the body and a sense of alienation from the material world.

For me movement is not about escaping reality but is a way of staying fully present with whatever I am experiencing and of embodying my responses to the world. As movement therapists, it's a requirement that we make a commitment to in-depth personal therapy before embarking on working with others therapeutically. It's received wisdom (and common sense) that we return to this engagement with personal therapy whenever it is necessary or supportive for us to do so. I would argue that a commitment to a personal movement practice is also essential and that this needs to be ongoing. How else are we to maintain an embodied connection to our own process as well as providing a secure embodied presence for our clients and students?

To continue, I am going to speak more about my approach to my personal movement practice and the role it plays in my life and work. I move both in the studio and in the natural environments where I live and work, primarily tidal sites on the Jurassic coast, the hill-tops above them and woodland on two hill-forts a few miles inland. An embodied kinaesthetic relationship to the natural world[4] is central to my practice. Both of the examples below take place in familiar coastal environments. More than simply the location in which the practice takes place, the environment is an essential partner with the moving body, the matrix within which the movement practice emerges, and is both teacher and therapist. Moving in the environment is informed by practice in the studio, and to a lesser extent vice versa, but what is elicited in the environment would not be generated in the same way in the studio.

I am writing experientially and autobiographically. I <u>need</u> to move. This is not about avoiding stillness, I value the depth and quietness of an established meditation practice. Moving is how I understand myself, how I understand what I am feeling, what is happening to me and how to be in the world. It is not an optional extra but a survival strategy, a way of staying sane, of healing myself, of untangling my limbs and my spine, my thoughts and my feelings, and of embodying and eventually integrating them. I am aware of the pitfalls of writing this personally in the arena of my professional practice but feel the need to speak out rather than sheltering behind the cloak of professional anonymity. While conscious of the need for a firm container with secure boundaries, there is a way in which this can become a form of hierarchy with the therapist masquerading as the sane one. I feel there is a place and a time for those of us who are elders within the profession to speak the truth of our experience, rather than revealing our professional practice while our personal experience remains shrouded in silence.

I am writing this at a particular time when those of us in the UK are emerging (or not) from our experience of 5 months of lockdown, the third period in 14 months. An unprecedented experience in most of our life-times and one which affected us all in a myriad of different ways and which has left a severe impact on our mental equilibrium as individuals, as a community and as a nation, which has yet to be fully examined.

The following are two pivotal moments in my practice in the environment both necessitated by the experience of lockdown. In May 2021, I experienced a day when my mental capacity to function healthily was in jeopardy. The warning signs had been building over a period of time but on this particular day the balance tipped. I was unaware of a specific trigger, rather that the mounting internal and external pressure had reached a crisis point. I experienced a severe narrowing down of my mental processes as if there was only a very small channel available to them. I found myself unable to think except in an extremely literal and linear fashion. I was unable to cope with anything unexpected, any change of plan or any new information coming in from elsewhere. I needed to know exactly what was happening and was unable to tolerate any sub-text or undercurrents. I had an acute and non-negotiable need to keep on my own track, stick to my plan. Within these very restricted parameters, I was able to function at least on a practical level.

Needless to say, relating in this state was virtually impossible. The mental constriction was accompanied by tension in my body. This acute mental rigidity was a desperate attempt to hang on to an illusion of control and stability in what was reflected in my dreams as a perilous sea with neither land nor boat in sight.

Fortunately, I had planned a day moving on the coast. This proved to be my boat and a life-saver. I went down to a wild rocky cove that I have spent time in and worked in over the past 40 years. I did not know where I was going to practise or what I was going to do. Ostensibly, I was preparing for a training group who had been unable to meet in person since the previous October and who would be arriving in a couple of weeks. The anxiety of re-entering a hall which I had last worked in over 18 months previously and complying with all the current restrictions added to the pressure I was experiencing.

Once on site, instead of going to areas which had attracted me recently, where streams of water from a large pool flow gently down between the rocks and pebbles to the sea, I found myself drawn to a liminal space of a very different character. Here, the rocks were being rapidly submerged by the wild incoming tide, accompanied by the roar of the waves in the open sea. Following my kinaesthetic intuition, rather than any conscious thought process, this proved to be exactly the environment I needed to practise in in order to re-stabilise. My body knew what needed to be done. I found myself stepping rhythmically from rock to rock, both wet and dry, sometimes getting my feet wet in an incoming wave, sometimes leaping, circling, changing direction, re-visiting, finding myself unexpectedly on the side of the rapidly filling pool, but returning again and again to close proximity with the wild incoming waves. I needed to be *there*. I realised later that the water, the sea, the waves and the wind were a precise antidote to the mental rigidity that had been restricting my capacity to think, to relate, to go with the flow. Standing on a large rock surrounded by wild water I was able to re-ground myself. Embracing the elements through Chi Gung, breathing and moving, I re-connected to my embodied presence, to the core of myself. Escaping the mental straitjacket that had been constraining me, I re-found stability and balance coupled with the ability to move from rock to rock, leaping between them like the synapses in the nervous system, making connections rather than compartmentalising, able to readily adjust to the changing surroundings as the tide came in, finding my way, choosing, turning, seeing the pathway through even as the world changed.

Afterwards, sitting drinking ginger tea on the pebble beach as the tide seeps ever closer, I bide my time before re-entering the society of other human beings and embracing my responsibilities. I know my place here, I feel at home. I savour the gift of re-connection with the natural world and with myself received at this fleeting moment in time. I know that my task as human being is to carry this with me as I re-enter relationship with others.

I know of no therapeutic intervention, however skilful, which would have returned me so fully and so pleasurably to my sense of self.

The second moment of movement practice which I would like to present took place just over two weeks later on a nearby coastal site of flat rock ledges and blue lias clay, interspersed with sandy plateaus, sea pools and rocky outcrops. I found myself unexpectedly practising alongside a group of experienced mentees as they engaged in their own movement practice. Attempting, responsibly and legally, to maintain an embodied practice for myself and in my professional work with others, in the months affected by recurrent lockdowns and constantly changing and unclear restrictions, had proved extremely challenging as an independent practitioner running a public programme. Immediately before the training group re-started, I experienced a state of heightened anxiety and doubt regarding my responsibilities and the decisions I was making. I was exhausted, furious and fed up of being emotionally and psychologically manipulated by a government of little integrity, with scant regard for the truth or the well-being of others, in a relationship which smacked more of coercive control than caring governance. Tactics, including bullying, deliberately heightening anxiety in an already frightened population, lying, emotional blackmail, excessive pressure to conform rather than making informed decisions, and encouraging the public to pressurise and control each other, for me evoked echoes of the Stasi in East Germany. As a result of this, our relationship to our body and our mental health has been severely compromised not only by the corona virus itself but also as a result of the political, media and medical responses to it.

In this political and personal context, my professional task was to continue to facilitate the mentoring programme embarked on in October 2020. Despite repeated postponements, I was determined to do so in person through an embodied process with the group rather than a pale attempt to replicate it online. The group reconvened four months later than scheduled, although we had kept in contact during the hiatus. After witnessing them for some time as they practised on site on the first day, I was surprised to find myself entering the site alongside them as my own movement practice erupted in response to all the aforementioned pressures. I found myself dancing like a banshee, the energy of outrage and fury coursing through my system in a bodily expression of the emotions I had been experiencing but without a specific narrative attached to them. The movements were strong, direct and jagged with extended arms and closed fists, strong legs lifted high, angular knees and elbows, kicks and punches. Indelicate, unapologetic movements claiming a lot of space accompanied by the roar of the waves and the crashes of sections of the cliff falling after excessive rain. I found myself offering a shout in response, my face contorted like a gargoyle. With contrary forces twisting my body, my limbs delineating lines in space, staccato movements and a strong flick of my extended arms it was clear: *There's no messing with me!*

This experience felt like a crucial expression, expelling the tension and craziness induced by the situation. Both an assertion of my own truth, of my right to occupy space and to breathe, and a refusal to agree with what was happening to us all. The expansiveness and scale of the site with the wide-open seascape and ancient, towering cliffs permitted a correspondingly dynamic release of energy and emotion without needing to direct it at another person or damaging myself or the environment. This full-bodied expression was experienced without re-inscribing the emotions concerned. A far cry from a Beckettian sense of resignation and inertia which periodically threatened to overwhelm me during lockdown.

On completion, I experienced a sense of having come back to myself, enabling me to be fully present with myself and with others.

These two examples demonstrate the unique capacity of the moving body as a therapeutic medium, a means to process feelings and experiences which cannot be as fully expressed through language sitting in a confined space (although they may be usefully explored and reflected upon) combined with the potential for an immediate and complete sense of resolution. As dance movement therapists and practitioners, we are uniquely placed to offer this opportunity to others. If, in addition, there is the capacity to work in relation to the wider material and natural environment, the potential of this practice may be both enhanced and magnified.

I invite you to go outside, to breathe, to open your senses and to begin to move. . . .

Notes

1 The terms 'check' and 'asking for guidance' are taken from Sumarah, a Javanese Meditation practice. See Romano (2013) for further information.
2 It is crucial when referring to work undertaken with clients that their anonymity is protected and that nothing is shared that may allow them to be identified. If it is possible to do so, their permission should be sought.
3 This image is derived from Suprapto Suryodarmo, a Javanese movement teacher with whom I trained intensively.
4 I am using the term 'natural' loosely, distinguishing it from the built environment, to refer to environments where elements such as earth, tree, rock and sea predominate.

References

Barks, C. (2006). *A year with Rumi*. New York: Harper One.
Romano, L. (2013). *Sumarah: Spiritual wisdom from Java*. Translated by Catherine Bearfield. Raleigh, NC: Lulu Press.

10 Being seen and seeing self

Explorations in the creative process in performance and therapy

Claire Burrell

Introduction: moving through the landscape

By holding creativity in relation to clinical practice, this chapter explores the entwining of my clinical and artistic embodied practice with vignettes and case examples from my work over the years. Describing how I have used photography and film to locate, consolidate and enhance embodied experience for both my clients and within my own creative process, I explore how to frame, make visible and witness embodiment; that is, ways to be seen and to see oneself. Perhaps to communicate personal narrative, to evidence the trace of life which has just passed, perhaps to see ourselves differently or to locate ourselves more fully as we negotiate ever-changing landscapes. Solnit (2005) reminds us that: 'The mind too can be imagined as a landscape [...] caverns, glaciers, torrential rivers, heavy fogs, chasms that open up underfoot, [...]. It's a landscape in which getting lost is easy and some regions are terrifying to visit' (53).

As Arts Psychotherapists, being able to adapt in the face of change is something we aspire to model in our work and creative processes both with our clients and with collaborators in our fields. However, losing your flow, your direction and indeed getting lost in the creating journey entirely remain perhaps integral parts of the experience for both the client and the therapist. Keeping sight of oneself is vital to journeying, and key to what I offer as a therapist.

Through my dance career and subsequent 20 years of clinical practice as a dance movement psychotherapist (DMP), the anchor of my work has been about locating embodied experience through dance and movement improvisation. The content of this chapter contributes to my ongoing exploration of transdisciplinary and cross-modality practice both as a therapist and artist / maker. By transdisciplinary, I refer to a creative process where two or more branches of inquiry become entwined in exploration, informing each other to the degree which transcends the traditional boundaries of their specific mediums in pursuit of a new way of working. However, cross-modality for me describes where two or more forms are side by side or are stages in a process, thus providing stages of exploration, in a layering and filtering experience

DOI: 10.4324/9781003222484-10

(Burrell & Cohen 2018) through sequential lenses. In this chapter, I bring forward the way in which I am moved by the organic nature of self-expression and the inseparability of form in the moment of creative inspiration.

Drawing on work offered to adult client groups both in the National Health Service (NHS) and in charity sector services, I will reflect on two photography exhibitions, both made with clients familiar with dance and movement therapy as a practice. 'These are My Hands' portrayed the expressive gestures of female asylum seekers and refugees, most of them caught in the limbo between what has been left behind and the uncertainty of how they might move their lives forward (Rova, Burrell & Cohen 2020). And 'Seeing Self' was an exploration of movement and photography, which, devised with a photographer from the onset, strove to give a sense of agency and control in the exploration of looking and seeing, encouraging a narrowing and widening of the gaze, whilst moving through changing environments. I will further illustrate how the theme of being seen is central to my professional identity with examples of my creative process, in particular the making of films, committing myself to being seen, in order to have a fuller understanding of myself. Throughout this writing, the content shared is with the permission of collaborators.

These are my hands

Since training as a DMP, I have been working with asylum seekers and refugees. I am curious about where this passion arises. Perhaps it stems largely from my own ten-year experience of living as a migrant in Europe, perhaps it links to the many small journeys of migration made by my ancestors. Early in my career I began offering DMP at Southwark Day Centre for Asylum Seekers, a charity organisation committed to addressing the breadth of support-needs faced by its client group. I explored different approaches to delivering DMP, offering separate groups for men and women and for a period of time worked as a Mental Health Support Worker, which helped to develop the work into a well-accessed, valued resource within the community.

Nestled within the busy day centre services, the women's DMP group offered drop-in sessions with open access. Over time, the group supported women from Eritrea, Sudan, Ethiopia, Iran, DR Congo, Ivory Coast, Syria, Kosovar, Albania, Algeria and many other places. Living in fragile temporary accommodation, surviving somewhere below the poverty line whilst awaiting Home Office outcomes for Asylum applications, made even the simplest of daily routines unpredictable and necessitated flexible access to sessions. The group held a space for many things; a place to rest on safe ground, a time to gather inner resources, resilience and a readiness to take the next steps, a place to mourn and remember all that had been left behind. It was a place to pause and bring forward stories, to build bridges across time and space, to speak old and new languages and to foster new ways of being.

I had become curious about the group's use of hand gestures, not only as communication in the absence of shared verbal language, but to express, recall and represent unique cultural traditions in the movements they committed to the space. Individual hand movements stood out boldly in emergent group dances like landmarks or flags from native traditions, brought forward perhaps as tools to navigate the present. The hand gestures and emerging movement metaphors (Bartal & Ne'eman 1993) enabled shared language to evolve, facilitating at times opportunity to express both common ground and the separateness of unique identity and differing perspectives. Often, the hand movements and gestures drew attention to a state of interruption, an experience of dislocation and separation but they also invited inquiry into future steps and into finding a way forward.

The vulnerable and fragile position refugee and asylum seekers face in the UK positions them as unheard, shrouded in invisibility, lost in silencing manoeuvres of political blanketing. Wanting to find a dignified way to value the group's collective expression and to enable them to be seen and see themselves within the wider local community, I became drawn to using photography, which like dance makes visible the expression of experiences difficult to put into words. Opportunity arose to participate in an event housed by a local museum, called 'Crossing Borders',[1] which sought to bring refugee organisations and their communities into focus. I began collaborating with a local photographer whose work as an artist and a writer was defined by a feminist ethos, advocacy of mental health issues and representation of marginalised communities, supported by the museum that agreed to produce the work. Choosing to focus the work on the women's hands gave a sense of safeguarding identity and I hoped this would allow the women to express themselves more freely.

The women were told about the idea of a photographic exhibition and invited to participate. Movement workshops offered over a few weeks provided space to deepen the exploration of the hand movements and each woman worked to decide upon the hand gesture, sculpt or metaphor they wished to have photographed. A confidential improvised studio space with adequate lighting was created with the photographer to work close-up with participants, in order to capture the gestures against a simple background. Because of the verbal language barrier, the photographer[2] worked with physical and gestural communication. She recalled how

> I showed and expressed my affect, I was moved by what I was being shown. I was informed by it. And I let them know this. There was also touch between us, we clasped hands, touched shoulders, there were many smiles and a sense of camaraderie. A sense of making something together.

The photographer also recalled how the women seemed keen to express themselves in front of the camera lens remembering how they seemed to 'throw their hands up into the light'.

'Going'

The women were also asked whether they would like to give a title or words to accompany their photographed gesture, which they did in several languages. One woman, who has given her consent to share her image and experience, used her fingers to express the sense of a walking pair of legs. She gave her walking fingers metaphor the title 'Going'. Suffering for a long time with debilitating depressive symptoms, migraines and joint inflammation, she had been diagnosed with a vitamin D deficiency and recommended to spend time outdoors.

> "Where are you going?" I remember asking in response to her gesture
> "I don't know," she replied, shrugging her shoulders, looking low.
> "Have you been going to the park?" I enquired.
> "To the park?" she replied, then slowly remembering the GP's recommendation
> "Not yet! But I will, now I have the legs!" she smiled walking her fingers.

Working with this image, both myself and the photographer were filled with overwhelming awareness of the power of this metaphor. Fear, flight and the immense effort carried forward were contained in the lightness of an apparently throwaway signal.

Reflecting on this project, my attention is drawn to the importance of offering choice within creative process; choice between engaging with implicit or explicit memory, between past and future narratives, memories of traumatising events or memories of ongoing survival. I felt the cross-modal practice had sustained a regulating environment enabling clients to 'experience greater safety and therefore an expanded capacity for tolerating both past and present experience' (Fisher 2017: 48) (Figure 10.1).

By approaching the process in different ways, choosing how to form and shape their experience and what to focus on in the present moment, each woman's photograph carried a unique, deep meaning. One of the women chose to have photographed her clicking fingers. This action, which produced a very distinctive sound, was linked directly to Iranian folk dance traditions. Another, who had always embodied her strength and resilience in the group, used the photograph to frame her disfigured, once broken little finger, which was a tender sharing of the less seen vulnerable part of self. The works represented women at differing stages of processing their experiences, journeys of flight, journeys of survival towards safety and well-being. Whilst one woman pushed her palms close in towards the camera, choosing the word 'Go', another made circles with her thumbs and index fingers and interlinked the two, calling her hand sculpture 'Love'.

For the exhibition, making visible the work whilst retaining anonymity enabled the group to be seen in a safe way. Many of the photographs were

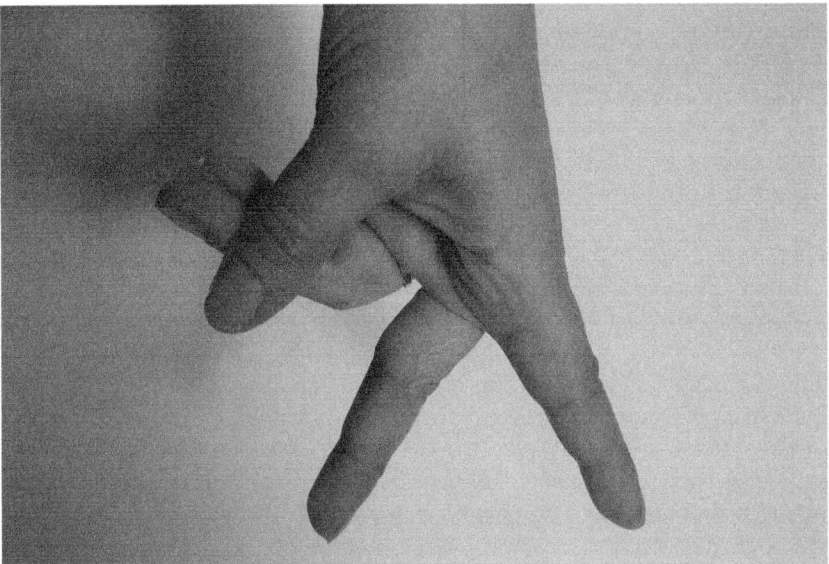

Figure 10.1 'Going'. Photograph by Nicola Field.

enlarged to poster size and stood out powerfully, with a sense of boundary intact. The work felt dignified; it held onto important landmarks and yet defined separation, indicating new ways forward. The women who visited their work in the exhibition seemed honoured and pleased with the results. I witnessed them as they met their images, curious about the way they positioned themselves in relation to the work: some stepping in closer, zooming in to see detail, some stepping back perhaps to take in the body of work or take more distance, some appeared more upright, quietly happy or shared a sense of achievement with their families.

It was reassuring to see them briefly dwell in a different space, a place of interaction with themselves, a place of interaction within the local community. The cross-modal practice enabled the women to make visible important landmarks, memories and intentions to be carried with them or left behind. Aesthetically, with hands disconnected from bodies and faces, the work portrayed a cut-off state, a sense of severed belonging. Initially, this triggered in me disappointment; I questioned whether I had failed to bring the women's experience into wholeness? In time, I came to consider this an integral layer of the work, but it led me to consider how this cross-modal practice represented the clients and made me curious to find a way of working which enabled more agency, control and engagement in the exploration of how we might choose to be seen.

Shifting positions and framing art

On the cusp of the millennium, my work became informed by the arts-based community, Studio Upstairs, whose work at that time was rooted largely in the therapeutic model of the radical Scottish psychiatrist R.D. Laing (Laing 1967). A founding member of the Philadelphia Association, concerned with understanding and improving the relief of mental suffering, Laing was famous for his psychiatric community project at Kingsley Hall, East London, where during the 1960s, radical residential approaches to treating people in mental health crisis were explored, allowing people to live freely with acute psychiatric illness, receiving no treatment they did not want.

My role at the Studio Upstairs involved working with the community's Performance Group, making collective work, which emerged from the long studio workshop days in the building's basement. Following the ethos that 'All life can be framed in Art' and as Art should be seen in the public arena, regular performances took place in the small black box theatre located in the then Diorama Arts Centre. Alongside Review style shows, full of auto-biographical content and poignant social political context, l recall also our version of William Shakespeare's 'The Tempest' and Lewis Carroll's 'Alice Through the Looking Glass'.

Making and performing with the group necessitated the taking of different positions. This exploration offered both a sense of stepping in and stepping out, swapping roles as if trying on the others' shoes, or by widening the lens further, shifting to take the more peripheral receptive position as the audience / witness. This inter-experience provided invaluable opportunity; in oscillating in and out of being seen and seeing others, we stimulated curiosity and conversation about our personal experiences and our experience of the behaviours of others (ibid).

The influence of this underpinning ethos has stayed with me over the years. As we work to serve marginalised communities, and those burdened by mental health illness, I feel that sharing artwork within a wider community, in a public context, has a place in the work we offer as arts therapies practitioners. I have a sense of widening the base, Not least through advocacy and the autonomy of self-representation but also through receptivity, the looking and witnessing which enables us to see our own experience reflected in the experiences of others, simultaneously meeting others and being met.

Seeing self – an exploration of movement and photography

Whilst working within an adult mental health NHS Arts Therapies Service, I was able to put forward again my interest in combining movement exploration with photography, envisaging this time a more integrated transdisciplinary process around the theme of *Seeing Self*. At the time (see: Seeing Self 2017), the service aimed to provide a summer project located at a partnership rehabilitation centre, which had space, resources and private access to an out-door garden. Within this context, a project was devised and co-led with a photographer who had existing experience in working within community mental health services. He felt that practising photography could be understood as a form of mindfulness, and connected this to dance movement and meditation. He described finding a sense of 'flow' when taking photos, which he linked both to an embodied presence and a sense of calming the mind, a relief from stress.

The project was designed as a series of one day workshops over five weeks, exploring the act of seeing and the experience of being seen, in order to create images that might represent self-experience and self-expression. As facilitators, we wanted to explore the possibility of integrating movement and photography as embodied exploration, as well as offering some minimum guidance in photography. Time was also allocated to viewing the images in an IT suite, enabling post-production enhancement and transformation. From the outset, the project worked towards an exhibition envisaging embodied images and photography as emotional communication, both to develop participants' confidence in being seen by others and to provide an opportunity to see their own work and to see themselves.

The workshops began with an experiential movement process offering improvised structures for working individually, in pairs and within the group context, focusing on the experience of seeing and being seen (e.g., moving in relation to narrowing and widening the gaze, or exchanging roles in being witnessed and witnessing).This encouraged both a shift between an internal and an external gaze and the potential to locate oneself relationally within a wider environment. The photographer,[3] moving with the group from the onset, tracked his own embodied experience, noting how his initial anxiety transformed into a more relaxed state 'increasing not just the interaction between my body and my mind but the connection with others in the group. I felt able to communicate not through words but through movement'.

Themes that had emerged in the movement exploration such as reflections and mirrors, revealing and concealing, were further explored as the photographer introduced the use of filters, reflective materials and a variety of lenses into the studio exploration. He described how the role of props in photography added character and context, particularly to portrait photography, where the intention might be to capture an aspect of the unique personality or the mood of an individual. As the group explored these elements, a layer of languaging was added, enhancing their capacity to see and speak about their experience, particularly when shooting self-portraits. The group explored changes of colour, the use of distortion, through filters and reflections of self, which enabled a shift of perspective or a sense of distancing.

The group then spent time working with cameras, collectively moving into accessible environments around the site. Time was spent working outdoors, first in the centre's garden, and as a later step, in the nearby park. Both the cameras and active looking state seemed to heighten a sense of questioning how far we could go. How far could we widen our lens whilst sustaining a sense of being in control? How far could we physically travel through the landscape?

Self(ie) control

Engaging with an image of oneself triggered anxiety in many members of the group; self-esteem was low, many suffered with negative body image and the impact of self-restricted isolative lifestyles due to past trauma. One member of the group had a public order restraint, another expressed paranoia in relation to how the images would be shared.

On a sunny day, several participants explored the idea of interacting with their own shadows, bringing into focus perhaps less visible parts of themselves. Some explored a sense of inhabiting their own shadow, improvising movement in relation to the image they saw, or exploring a range of qualitative expressions. Capturing the shadow images as selfies enhanced their sense of control and autonomy. One such photograph shows a figure stepping into their own shadow: the shadow of the author of the image points intentionally forward, their foot visible within the shadow. There is a clarity in what has been framed and a sense of ownership of the moment for 'unlike any other visual image, a photograph is not a rendering, an imitation or an interpretation of its subject, but actually a trace of it' (Berger 2013: 51).

The experience of interpersonal trauma can teach us to become invisible, making seeing ourselves exceptionally difficult. Choosing to represent a part of the self which is experienced as not there or just a shadow, beginning to embody this, perhaps not yet able to bring the parts fully together but to tolerate a sense of them in one place at the same time, is to question how much of myself can be here right now? Borzello (2016) explores how self-portraits have developed from the simple, 'this is what I look like' to the more complicated, 'this is what I believe in'. The Seeing Self photography work encouraged further framing of identity: 'this is how I experience myself' and 'this is how I can tolerate being seen by others'.

At all stages of the process, freedom of choice was prioritised, and participants were encouraged to consider what would be framed, what would be deleted or retained and later in post-production, what might be transformed or edited. As images were considered, a process which took several additional meetings in the IT suite, the idea of publicly sharing the work was continuously discussed. Considering individually what work to commit to the exhibition, to take its place in a collective body of work, was a huge step for the group. I felt strongly that the work should be hung outside of the hospital in a space accessible to a wider public, and an arts-based local mental health charity, with open gallery space, was chosen to house the work.

Participants had engaged in the project with curiosity and creativity which seemed enhanced by the embodied sense of a focusing lens and the autonomous sense of control the photographic collaboration had been enabled.

Their arrival at the Private View event of the exhibition was honest and courageous, as anxiety and nerves prevailed.

I found myself pacing through the exhibition a few times... each time zooming in to a different detail or noticing different themes and stories.... I was struck by the integrity of the work, the professionalism in presenting the material and the flow of movement, image and narrative running through (Seeing Self 2017).

I was pleased how visitors to the exhibition experienced the movement in the images and described something more, akin to what Reason (2012) refers to as 'those moments when we do not just perceive within a photograph that something moved or was about to move but begin to internalise or be affected by that perception of movement' (247).

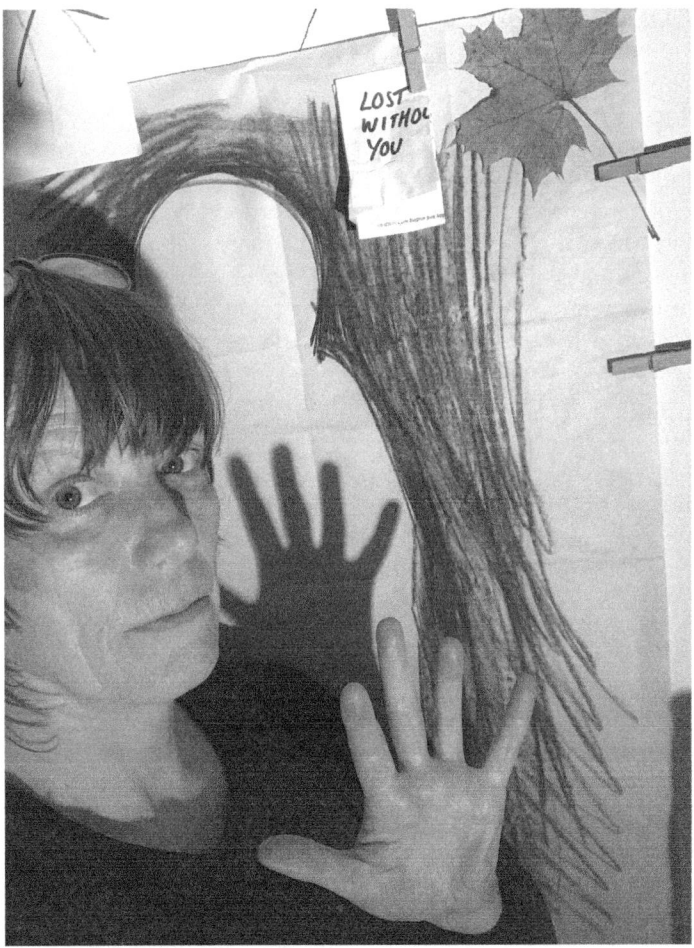

Figure 10.2 'Lost without you'. Photograph by Claire Burrell.

For many there were challenges; for some physical hurdles and for others control of personal boundaries, particularly when relating to others, stayed in focus. Working with photography allowed the group to communicate something of that inner dialogue, and give it a visible, authentic trace. It allowed the more vulnerable parts of self to emerge and be seen.

Continued surrender

There is much to be considered by the therapist who travels unknown paths with their clients. Resources need safeguarding, nurturing and replenishing. Navigation tools, maps and recognisable landmarks enable us to steer our course, but we must be able to relocate and return to self. That embodied sense of knowing my way back home, (Lyengar 2005; Papadopoulos 2015) is what I connect to in order to support the clients' way back. It is a regulating process anchored in my nervous system and it needs to be regularly attuned to. To do this, I need a set of flexible embodied tools which allow me to dwell in my own frame and experience so that I might see myself more clearly. It needs to be an honest process where the parts of myself can come together.

Yoga, meditation and movement improvisation, particularly in the natural landscape, each provide valuable frames through which the cultivation of both internal and external gazes support me to look more clearly. Engaging in my own creating / making process provides a self-regulating frame that holds me as I search and reveal. I have been involved in the making of three short films, each in their own way an inquiry into how trauma is held, carried and released in the body, each capturing movement which is improvised and biographical. Two of them capture recovery journeys following life-threatening illness, documenting lived narrative. In doing so, it has become clear to me 'that the therapist in making their own artwork pursues a vital process of self-care' (West 2018: 236).

The short film *Continued Surrender* grew from my desire to map and make visible the oscillation of repeated trauma patterning, albeit in the throes of everyday mayhem. I was interested to make visible the juxtaposition of what compels us to continue and what enables us to stop and to yield. The dancer was invited to identify areas of somatic discomfort which we mapped and traced as trauma lines through the body's default pathways. Connecting to birthing, illness in pregnancy, parenting and family dynamics, the dancer began to articulate her sense of embodied holding, embodied memory. An antidote or a counterbalance was then explored, emergent moments of release, of suspended time, merging with the landscape in a resignation of the need to come to ground. As we discussed the state of surrender in the work, the dancer questioned the proposed title for the work; she told me, 'I'm not giving up, Claire, I'll never give up'. Her resilience is arguably what stands out for me in the work as a whole. And of course, in this, I see myself.

Continued capers

During the 2020–2021 coronavirus pandemic, what began as a plan for a creative residency for a group of artists became an on-line lockdown trans-disciplinary survival project. Retaining its original project title, 'Capers', the work became both an expression of empathy and an umbilical cord of connectivity, strong enough to allow for the exploration of the restricted movement, isolation and loss which dominated these unprecedented times. As many of us have discovered, selecting the gallery view on video conferencing calls facilitates seeing each other contemporarily existing side by side, providing opportunity to be seen and see oneself simultaneously albeit with a few WiFi delays and frame freezes. Often our creative process was navigated by a set of rules and an agreed set of materials, enabling familiar landmarks whilst cohabiting in a virtual place, in a new era. One of the 'rules' in each session was to capture a selfie (Figure 10.2).

Conclusion

I acknowledge that my work is enabled, influenced and co-created in the relational process of working with others; arts therapists and artists from diverse disciplines and by the clients who courageously step forward into the potential of the creative therapy space.

In this chapter, I have reflected on how cross-modal and transdisciplinary processes, integral to the way I work as a dance movement psychotherapist, can offer tools, structures and lenses through which to illuminate our embodied experiences, supporting our clients and ourselves to see more clearly. I have discussed how photography and films provide habitable structures, modes to both frame and transcend the boundaries of our embodied experience and provide a sense of tangible holding as we move through landscapes where getting lost is easy.

Making the work of marginalised communities visible, making mental health visible, de-stigmatisation, and exploring collaborative approaches in therapy have remained the essential components of my work and largely what moves me. I have highlighted how framing art in the public arena can be an integrating experience, facilitating a sense of taking one's place in the wider community. Furthermore, I offer the reader a sense of how this might be sensitivity achieved, by giving agency, choice and control in the process of sharing work and committing to being seen.

I encourage continuous and curious investigation of the tools and resources available to therapists so that they might adapt frames of reference to support their clients to feel seen. Furthermore, I advocate that therapists commit, within their own personal exploration and unique creative practices, to being seen and thus seeing themselves in ways that enable them to continue to move through the therapeutic landscape and provide a stable source of regulated energy to their clients. I have drawn on my sense of how life continuously requires me to re-attune, refocus and reframe my perspective. I have reflected on how nurturing vulnerability, bringing it forward in our creative exploration, can enhance our capacity to see ourselves with compassion and awareness, vital to our self-care and longevity.

In my work, I try to remain aware and in contemplation of how much of ourselves shapes the act of seeing and frames how we choose to be seen by considering the obscured view of positions we might hold and, from the other side of the lens, I ask how we experience and tolerate the vulnerability of exposure and, I remain curious as to how, in the midst of glaciers and torrential rivers, reflection will meet us.

Writing this chapter, recalling images from the entanglement of my clinical, artistic and embodied practice, serves to relocate me to the present moment. It brings a sense of perspective, a refocusing, perhaps a synthesis, that brings clarity and reassurance in preparation of moving forward once again.

Thanks to all my creative collaborators, particularly to those whose work is discussed here: Alexis Matila, Nicola Field and Emma Texidor.

Notes

1 The Horniman Museum located in Forest Hill, London, annually hosts its "Crossing Borders" event, celebrating the creative achievement of local refugee and asylum seeker communities.
2 Nicola Field was the photographer and collaborator for the "These are My Hands" project and exhibition.
3 Alexis Matilla was the photographer and collaborator for the "Seeing Self – an exploration of movement and photography" project and exhibition.

References

Bartal, L. & Ne'eman, N. (1993). *The metaphoric body: guide to expressive therapy through images and archetypes.* London: Jessica Kingsley Publishers.
Berger, J. (2013). *Understanding a photograph, edited and introduced by Geoff Dyer.* London: Penguin Books.
Borzello, F. (2016). *Seeing ourselves: women's self-portraits.* London: Thames and Hudson.
Burrell, C. & Cohen, M. (2018). Moving colour: combining dance movement psychotherapy and art psychotherapy in a NHS community women's group. In Colbert, T. & Bent, C. (eds.) *Working across modalities in the arts therapies: creative collaborations,* Oxon & New York: Routledge, pp. 15–29.
Fisher, J. (2017). *Healing the fragmented selves of trauma survivors.* New York: Routledge.
Iyengar, B.K.S. (2005). *Light on life.* London: Roledale Books.
Laing, R.D. (1990). *The politics of experience and the bird of paradise.* (3rd edition). London: Penguin Books.
Papadopoulos, N. (2015). The body as home. *E-Motion Quarterly ADMPUK,* XXV (3), pp. 4–7.
Reason, M. (2012). Photography and the representation of kinaesthetic empathy. In Reynolds, D. & Reason, M. (eds.) *Kinaesthetic empathy In creative and cultural practices,* Chicago: Intellect, pp. 237–256.

Rova, M., Burrell, C. & Cohen, M. (2020). Existing in-between two worlds: supporting asylum seeking women living in temporary accommodation through a creative movement and art intervention. *Body, Movement and Dance in Psychotherapy*, 15 (3), pp. 204–218.

Seeing Self (2017). Seeing Self exhibition comments book.

Solnit, R. (2005). *A field guide to getting lost*. New York: Viking Books.

West, J.D. (2018). *Art therapy in private practice*. London: Jessica Kingsley.

11 Finding my way home

An embodied journey to building an inclusive dance community

Juliet Diener

Introduction

Dance has always been part of my lived bodily experience. From the earliest memories of dancing around the dinner table of my childhood home, to when I wore my first tutu and took centre stage. Dance has been core to how I express myself, and now how I understand myself, others and the world around me. Speaking to dance teachers from various dance genres, at the International Summer School hosted by the Imperial Society of Teachers of Dancing in August 2019, I asked the question, 'Why do you dance?' 'The responses were emotional, heartfelt and often embedded in childhood memories, with the overriding expression being that dance brings joy and allows dancers to be themselves' (Diener 2020: 20). For many, dance was where they felt most at 'home' and offered not just a physical experience but a connection with emotionality. Identifying the ability for dance to express an inner world that doesn't always have language echoes the words by Martha Graham, an influential American dancer and choreographer who expressed 'Dance is the hidden language of the soul' (Graham 1985: 1). The transformative power of dance was acutely experienced by the dance teachers attending the summer school, and so too, influences my creative journey. My answer to the same question comes from a research journal entry dated February 2020:

> I feel complete when I do. That all my parts fit together to create a story-My story. I can't not and when I don't dance, I don't feel fully me. I feel centered when I do. I become a better version of myself.

The completeness and centering which I describe gives me a sense of coming home in my body. Home, meaning a place within, of acceptance, connecting, knowing and creativity. As I write and reflect on these words, my body feels grounded, rooted and centered. My personal story has been the catalyst of the creation of my professional home, icandance. icandance aims to make dance possible for all, offering a creative therapeutic community, with the vision of celebrating the abilities of disabled children and young people to enrich all lives through dance and performance.

DOI: 10.4324/9781003222484-11

Established in September 2006 and registering as a charity in 2010, ican-dance takes a pioneering interdisciplinary approach, drawing on Dance Movement Psychotherapy, dance and education techniques. The approach places disabled children and young people centre stage and challenges per-ceptions of disability, through dance. It offers each dancer the opportunity to explore their experience of being in the world through creative expression, skill development and nurturing relationships.

Each week, we work with on average 120 children and young people aged 4–25 years old with varied learning, physical, social and emotional needs, in-cluding complex medical conditions. We offer direct support for each dancer, their families and professionals within the wider community. Whilst we are an established inclusive dance community, the process of shaping icandance started with 'me', which led to a discovery of the other, which I describe as 'you' and to eventually shape an 'us', through establishing a community. In this chapter, I will share this journey with reference to embodied processes and the dancers who helped me build the community.

Me

'The question we pose to our clients and patients, "what brings you here?", must also be asked of ourselves' (Adams 2014: 16). I embody the concept of 'here' feeling grounded and rooted with a sense of centre. The word 'here' represents various parts of me. First, a physical place as a South African now living in London. Second, an intellectual exploration of the shaping of the approach I created at icandance. Finally, my emotional 'here', as I acknowl-edge my very core experiences that have shaped the values which underpin my work.

As I begin to write, my body wants to move the story and a natural re-sponse arises as I hear the statement ring in my ears, 'You create a tribe'. As I write I embody my tribeswoman which feels grounded, wide and firmly weighted, whilst open, welcoming and strong, a gatherer of people, a collec-tor of stories, a community builder, a curator of values. When I embody the word tribeswoman, it evolves into community and is circular, symbolic of the tribeswoman sitting by the fire, waiting for her people to gather after a long day apart.

The fire is the meeting point where everyone gathers to receive warmth, nourishment and connection. There is a place for everyone, and all have a role to play in the shaping of the tribe. As I reflect on the metaphor of the tribeswoman, the renowned novel by Chinua Achebe (1958) *Things fall apart* comes to my consciousness. Whilst trying to be a good tribesman Okonkwo, from the Nigerian Igbo community, finds himself conflicted between the enemies outside of his tribe i.e., the white man/colonisers, and the demons he finds within. I read this book at university whilst pursuing a degree in teach-ing, noting it was the first time I had read any literature written by a black author. The novel shares the unravelling of the tribal values of the Igbo tribe, as the white colonisers and missionaries arrive to 'save' them, change them and ultimately break the tribe: 'He (meaning the white colonisers) has put a knife on the things that held us together and we have fallen apart' (Achebe 1958: 135). The tribal fire was extinguished, their values disregarded and differences quashed. Their 'otherness' was not welcome.

Brons (2015) in his paper entitled 'Othering, an Analysis' offers insights on definitions of othering. Brons cites cultural geographer Crang, who describes othering as 'a process (...) through which identities are set up in an unequal relationship' (Crang cited in Brons 2015: 70). He continues to summarise Crang's words that, 'Othering thus sets up a superior self/in-group in contrast to an inferior other/out-group, but this superiority/inferiority is nearly always left implicit' (Crang cited in Brons 2015: 70).

The superiority/inferiority otherness was the backdrop to my childhood and was explicit in the apartheid years of South Africa. Apartheid translated from the Afrikaans language means 'apartness' and was introduced as law in 1948 by the Nationalist Party, to segregate people of different ethnicities, specifically black and white people (History.com Editors 2020). As I write these words, I feel the horror of this story in my body, twisting round and round in the pit of my stomach. I lived it, witnessed it and took part in it. The othering was acted out through housing, schooling, transport and relationships, to keep black and white people apart. Fear fuelled apartheid, and the inability to see black and white as part of the same tribe. The human tribe. The 'us' and 'them' phenomenon was fed as truth to the white South Africans, masking humanity and applying beastly attributes to the freedom fighters. The divide of 'otherness' poisoned us all and apartheid ruled as differences warred on each other in the streets, and conflict rose in the homes. Taking a socially constructivist view, my initial understanding of community was deeply scarred by this personal experience of a segregated community, which influenced me to be a tribeswoman who brings people together, rather than driving them apart.

Otherness and segregation were no longer tolerated as the outsider, Nelson Mandela, proved to us all that anything is possible as the once prisoner became president of the country. The raging external conflicts inflicted by apartheid felt internalised, as I sat with an internal conflict, that the prisoner was now the president and the messages which accompanied my childhood were wrong. But unlike the Igbo tribe, the very falling apart of what South Africa once was enabled a new beginning. My cultural and ethical paradigms significantly shifted and whilst unsettling, it felt liberating. Ponterotto (following Dilethy) notes that 'every 'lived experience' [author's emphasis] occurs within a historical social reality' (Ponterotto 2005: 129). My lived experience of this historical moment was transformative, as I witnessed the power of change, acceptance and inclusion as Nelson Mandela took his place as president of South Africa, welcoming a divided nation to gather at the tribal fire of forgiveness and reconciliation. My loathing of exclusion, othering and segregation began with apartheid but wasn't found only there.

Moving to London, I met the ideology of inclusion but soon discovered the challenges in which this ideology was rooted.

You

As I reach beyond my internal process I embody 'you'. I reach out and step towards new beginnings spring boarded by experiences from my past as my body feels light and full of flow, allowing me to reach forward with knowing and anticipation. Teaching in London was enticing, and I was excited by my first introduction to inclusion.

The Warnock report, chaired by Baroness Warnock and published in 1978, was a comprehensive review of special educational needs and disabilities, commissioned by the UK government (Webster 2018). The report,

> changed education and how far it now underpins much of what we do when it comes to SEND (special educational needs and disability). This report was, and remains, relevant because it marked a fundamental shift in discourse on special needs and disability, and accelerated progress towards inclusive approaches to education.
>
> (para.13)

The UK's approach to inclusion was ground-breaking and hoped to eradicate the divide of 'othering' created previously in society. Working within inclusive settings, I soon realised that whilst the report and subsequent 1981 Education Act (Webster 2018) offered a new way of thinking about disability, it required resources, a shift in community thinking and a change in language and expectations. Over 40 years on from the report, whilst there have been fundamental shifts in inclusive practice and societal acceptance of difference, the inclusion revolution continues. Frizell, a dance movement psychotherapist and parent of a disabled adult, speaks of being, 'trapped between the theory of inclusion and the painful lived reality of exclusion' (Frizell 2021: 3–4). This lived reality was evident in my practice and too became my own lived experience.

Holding qualifications as a ballet teacher, special educational needs teacher and dance movement psychotherapist, I found myself shape-shifting across London in various settings, client groups and roles. The splitting of my professional practice began to feel limiting, and the qualities of each role merged internally and impacted on my professional outlook. At times they collided causing friction, which slowly developed into fusion. I found myself exploring connections between cognition, emotion and motion. Finding these meeting points of the thinking, feeling, moving body allowed me to further explore, bringing my dance, education and therapy pathways together. The fusion led to integration of my professional worlds, as I sought out new emotionally informed ways of meeting the needs of children and young people with disabilities. I began to explore shaping a unique approach as delivered at my newly founded charity, icandance.

Becoming a parent arrived at a time of professional beginnings, as my child's birth collided with the registration of the charity. I became a parent overnight to two, as the charity and my child were born and both needed me more than I had predicted. Unexpected illness led to insight and whilst I was focused on the isolation, loss and grief experienced by parents with disabled children, with whom I worked, I realised I was not immune to such feelings. Whilst I apply an integrated approach at icandance, it is the very integration and application of my skills in my personal life that has enabled me to connect to the families in the icandance community. I have developed a deeper understanding of the lived experience of disability, isolation and exclusion. This strengthened my resolve to build an inclusive community.

Us

As I write, I centre my body to find my weight and feel grounded. I pause to breathe, to connect with my inner voice and to find a central point of calm. My arms are at my sides, resting gently, but not limp, and my feet are firmly rooted with a softness in my knees and a strength in my core reaching outwards into my back, shoulders and neck. My body is part of the process and not separate from it, and together my thinking, feeling, moving body continues to shape my journey. I embody the experience of 'us'.

Having experienced the divide which difference can cause, I sought to create a 'home' where all are equally valued and where those with disabilities are celebrated for their positive contribution to society. I established icandance to offer a creative, therapeutic community for families with lived experience of disability. The charity nurtures creativity, learning and well-being through weekly dance experiences. Alongside our weekly group icandance sessions, we offer our community of disabled dancers additional pathways of progression to further enhance their learning and development. Our Young Ambassadors group and supported volunteer roles for our Alumni offer our dancers opportunities to share their views to guide the charity, develop confidence through hosting events and nurture leadership and advocacy skills. Dancers with greater independence take part in our youth performance group, iam Dance Company. The company's weekly session is a space to explore choreography and offers additional performance opportunities to challenge society's perceptions of disability and dance.

To further support disabled children and young people's emotional health, we offer individual Dance Movement Psychotherapy sessions. These sessions offer young people a creative space to explore and understand their experiences in the world alongside the support of a skilled professional. The therapist works creatively to address anxieties and fears, and seeks opportunities to develop communication, confidence and overall enhanced well-being. We cater for parents through our Parent Therapy Groups, offering parents a supported space to reflect with other parents on the joys and challenges of parenting a disabled child. These groups are facilitated by experienced Dance Movement Psychotherapists.

icandance's specialist approach considers how a dancer moves, thinks and feels, with the latter being the foundation step to any dancer's arrival in a session. The approach is relational, transformative and deeply rooted in building a collaborative, creative and therapeutic community. It is multi-layered, interdisciplinary and infinitely subtle yet specific in intent and process. Embedded in the principles of Dance Movement Psychotherapy, we focus on how a child or young person feels before we focus on what they do, and how this is then expressed through the body, and witnessed by others. Both the disabled dancer and their non-disabled dance partner are changed by what they create. It is this creative shift that forms the foundation of our inclusive dance community. We work with the body in the here and now, while noting the presence of experiences that shape the story being told through the dance created.

This is formed relationally, as the dancer and dance partner mutually create, connect and share. Relationships are built through embodied therapeutic tools, which support the dancer emotionally to then be challenged physically and intellectually. This is then shared through performances and various community events which invite the wider community to join in the celebration of difference and to be changed by the experience. The transformation of such a performance was experienced by one of our dancers, Ella.[1]

Ella joined icandance when still in primary school, desperately longing to fulfil her dream of being a dancer. Having been told it was not possible for her due to being born with Cerebral Palsy, Ella and her family were determined to find a place where her disability was not seen as a barrier to her pursuing a dream. Finding icandance offered Ella an opportunity to find a place where she could develop in skill, creativity and emotional strength to overcome not only the physical challenges to dancing but fears and anxieties too.

Ella and some of her dancing peers are part of an inclusive leadership group at icandance called the Young Ambassadors, who are secondary school aged members of the icandance community. Their role is to be the voice of the young people of icandance and to offer guidance, ideas and reflections to the executive management of the charity. I met with the group in October 2021 and asked their thoughts on the importance of dance. This is what group members Ella and Tammy shared (Young Ambassadors recorded meeting, October 12, 2021):

> Dance can unleash a different side of you. You can unleash parts of you that you didn't know were there. There is a part of dance that is about the physicality as you realise different body parts that perhaps you haven't used as much but it also helps you to unleash the thoughts you didn't know existed in your mind but they do, and you find them through dancing.
>
> Ella (icandance dancer)

> I love dance and recognise its value because it's what connects us. There are so many different languages and through dance is a way everybody

can understand each other because emotions are shown in the same way. Dance is just so vital with communication and portraying emotion and connecting with different cultures and different people.

Tammy (icandance peer volunteer)

Ella was able to fulfil a dream when she was 14 years old as she performed in a theatre in London in July 2017 with two professional dancers. The choreography was created working with her body and her needs, together shaping a new way of moving with her professional dance partners. She focused on her strengths and had to develop her courage as she allowed herself to be lifted by the male dancers as part of the performance. Together, all three dancers created a new story which moved the audience to their feet and confirmed for us all of what is possible when inclusive practice meets creative resources and is supported by community belief. Inclusion offers a bringing together and re-moulding. However, I propose that inclusion be the act of building together, brick by brick, step by step, from the ground up to create a meeting place where everyone belongs, and all needs are catered for. Communities adapt 'to people rather than people having to adapt to them' (Jarrett 2020: 10).

Whilst I write this chapter, we are still living with the COVID-19 pandemic where unpredictability has become commonplace, requiring all of us to adapt, shape and rethink day-to-day living choices. Being adaptable, even at a moment's notice, is familiar to any family living with a child or young adult with disabilities. The ability to be flexible is central to responding inclusively to the needs of those with disabilities. The pandemic has forced me to re-evaluate what it means to offer an inclusive, creative community.

New ways of working and a redefinition of what is important have become an organisational and personal imperative as we have continued to strive to meet the needs of the icandance community during difficult circumstances. While the pandemic forced us to revisit our way of working, the relationships we fostered throughout it were rooted in existing partnerships. It became evident that, because we had built and maintained nurturing relationships before the crisis unfolded, we could support families at a time when they were feeling most vulnerable and isolated. Considering the needs of all members of society should never be a crisis response. It should be part of day-to-day practice as everyone, regardless of need, is welcomed and valued as an equal member of society.

Conclusion

As I come to the end of my journey in this chapter, my body surges with energy and vigour burning with a desire to continue to evolve the story of icandance as the charity is shaped by the community it serves. As I conclude, my movements are continuous, busy and circular as I dance around the tribal fire knowing I am not alone in the dance or the journey. My body moves freely, wildly yet controlled and purposeful as my feet stamp to the rhythm of the tribal beat. I embody the word community and feel ready.

From the beginning embers of otherness, experiences of isolation, mothering, tribal gatherings and the unwavering belief in possibilities, fanned the flame of icandance. A philosophical home representing the values I've gathered along my embodied journey, as well as the physical experience of creating a community for all to meet. Whilst creating the logo for my charity, I wanted it to emulate the colours of a burning fire (visit www.icandance. org.uk to view the logo). The fire of a tribal gathering, the fire of the passion burning inside of me and the fire I wanted others to see, as the values it represented lit up the darkest divide and offered an invitation which read: 'All are welcome here'. Dance offers us the creativity to be able to adapt, shape and respond to the needs of all in a manner that is accepting, uplifting and unifying. Applying an embodied, creative, psychotherapeutic approach within an inclusive dance community enriches dancers and their family's quality of life as perceptions of disability are challenged, creativity, learning and wellbeing are nurtured, and families are supported to explore dance and embodied processes as a tool for everyday living.

The meeting place of my experiences is an internalised tribal fire, where gathering together we, 'imagine disability differently' and explore 'difference itself as an opportunity to discover new ways of participating in communities' (Frizell 2021: 15). As I have shared through this chapter, this started with 'me', shaped by the influence of 'you', i.e. experiences outside myself, which have led me to reach out to create an 'us' community where all are accepted, invited and belong. With the moving, thinking, feeling body as core to building relationships, icandance offers a community which celebrates difference. I continue to name its various components, research its impact on families and witness its evolution as the charity responds to the lived experience of its community. Finally, I hope to continue to build a community where belonging is embraced, difference is celebrated, and creative bodily experiences are key to building and supporting inclusive communities.

Note

1 Consent has been given by those quoted in this chapter and pseudonyms are used.

References

Achebe, C. (1958). *Things fall apart. In The African trilogy.* London: Penguin.

Adams, M. (2014). *The myth of the untroubled therapist.* London/New York: Routledge.

Brons, L. (2015). Othering, an analysis. *Transcience*, Vol. 6 (1), pp. 69–90.

Diener, J. (2020). Why do we dance? Dance - The International Magazine of The Imperial Society of Teachers of Dancing, Issue 488, January- April 2020, pp. 20–21.

Frizell, C. (2021). Learning disability imagined differently: an evaluation of interviews with parents about discovering that their child has down's syndrome. *Disability & Society*, Vol. 36 (10), pp. 1574–1593.

Graham, M. (1985). Martha Graham reflects on her art and a life in dance. The New York Times on the web, March 31st, Section 2, p. 1. Retrieved from https://www.nytimes.com/1985/03/31/arts/martha-graham-reflects-on-her-art-and-a-life-in-dance.html.

History.com Editors (2020). Apartheid. Retrieved from https://www.history.com/topics/africa/apartheid.

Jarrett, S. (2020). *Those they called idiots. The idea of the disabled mind from 1700 to the present day.* London: Reaktion Books.

Ponterotto, J.G. (2005). Qualitative research in counselling psychology: a primer on research paradigms and philosophy of science. *Journal of Counselling Psychology,* Vol. 52 (2), pp. 126–136.

Webster, R. (2018). Why the Warnock report still matters today. TES. Retrieved from https://www.tes.com/magazine/archived/why-warnock-report-still-matters-today.

12 Dancing in the kitchen

Using creativity and embodiment to promote a decolonising approach to psychotherapy

Archana Ballal

'I'm ok thanks, I don't need therapy…. there's nothing wrong with me' is a phrase I hear so often during initial sessions with my clients. These clients have been identified as in need of psychotherapeutic intervention by professionals supporting them in two separate contexts in which I have worked as a therapist. The first context is the young person who is a Care Leaver and the second is the young person in prison custody at a Youth Offending Institution (YOI). These are young people between the ages of 16 and 21. I increasingly question how the systems in which I work evoke feelings in my clients of something being inherently *wrong* with *them*. In this chapter, I share some aspects of my work as a British-Indian, female Dance Movement Psychotherapist and I explore how a *creative* approach can begin to address some of the barriers to accessing therapy for these young people who find themselves on the margins of society. By not only working creatively in session, but also thinking creatively about how to challenge ethically some boundaries of the psychotherapeutic work to offer a more genuinely accessible therapy space, that is a *decolonised* space. I explore how the use of creativity and embodiment can promote a decolonising approach to psychotherapy, to enable a positive, supportive and meaningful intervention which does not further exclude. Here, I write about this from my perspective, protecting confidentiality in composite illustrations of case examples as I strive to represent the work and investment of my clients respectfully and sensitively.

Sepälä et al. (2021) define decolonising research methods as a 'process or practice that actively seeks to transform colonial and Eurocentric research practices based on hegemonic Western epistemologies by repositioning the research participants at the centre of the research process and developing alternative ways of engagement to support their perspectives and interests…the process of decolonising does not start with the "other", but rather trying to decolonise oneself and transform one's practices' (6–7).

Applying this to psychotherapy practice, I aim to reposition the client at the centre of the therapy work to address the power structures in place, ultimately enabling my clients to hold a more empowered and leading role, whilst utilising creativity and working with embodiment to foster engagement from their perspectives and interests. I also hold awareness of the racial trauma that

DOI: 10.4324/9781003222484-12

is held at an embodied level, including the intergenerational trauma passed down in non-verbal and unconscious processes. Holding in mind what Ellis (2021) describes as a visceral experience of racism, in the 'ever present threat to the physical boundaries of our bodies and threat of physical violence' (57), as well as the impact of status and power on bodies, Ellis notes how higher status bodies receive higher degrees of safety, more rights and more access to resources. In the race construct, the body of colour will have a lifetime of exclusion and coercion when comparing it with the white body (176).

Centring an embodied approach to psychotherapy enables a deeper acknowledgement and therefore exploration of the impact on bodies of colour, allowing a client to build trust in their own bodily responses and acknowledging how these factors contribute to interactions with others, and in engagement with the therapy space.

Key to hold in mind is the intersectionality (Crenshaw 1989) of the overlapping factors which combine to shape a young client's experience of the world. That is, the experience of being othered and discriminated against, through the intersections of, for example, race, gender and factors of social exclusion. The intersections present in the two separate clinical environments mentioned above cannot be ignored. Over a quarter of the adult prison population has previously been in care (HMPPS 2019), and the Youth Justice Board (2015) response to the independent review chaired by Lord Lamming highlights a wide range of factors that contribute to the number of care-experienced children (i.e., children who have had experience of the care system or of being looked after by the Local Authority at any point in their lives, for any length of time) who offend, being more than double the number of children from the general population. A high proportion of these young people are people of colour, from Black, Asian and Minority Ethnic backgrounds, as they are overrepresented in both the care and criminal justice systems (Lammy 2017; Lensvelt et al. 2021).

Research has highlighted that young people at risk of social exclusion find it harder to access support for their mental health. Those at high risk of social exclusion are frequently care-experienced, are from households where family conflict and poverty are present, are those who have had poor school attendance and those from minority ethnic communities (Youth Access 2002). The perceived stigma of needing support for mental health issues is compounded by these young people navigating systems of marginalised or excluded groups, due to being care-experienced or having a criminal record. Some report expressing concern that accessing support for their mental health may add to 'existing feelings of public misperception and stigmatisation at being care experienced' (Sanders 2020). Young people in youth offending institutions are often preoccupied by the burden of having a criminal record and how this will impact their prospects upon release; they often share that they do not wish to carry another label of needing support with their mental health.

Vulnerability to mental health issues is further pronounced in these young people who are from minority backgrounds, considering the experience of racism and discrimination, and the impact racism can contribute to mental ill health (Alleyne 2005; Williams 2018). It is important to acknowledge that there are also additional barriers to accessing mental health support for these young people. Ellis (2011) cites Lennox Thomas, who notes:

> There is history there. Like all institutions of power and authority, Psychiatry has been wielded against minorities. Psychotherapy has been subsumed under the heading of Psychiatry and there is no doubt that this institution has been seen as dangerous and untrustworthy.
>
> (190)

Lowe (2014) also articulates that as psychotherapy is still a predominantly white middle class profession, beliefs are reinforced of it being only for white middle class clients.

The following case vignettes aim to demonstrate how centring a creative and embodied approach can address some of these very real barriers and power imbalances, create safety, regulation and group cohesion, enabling clients to explore not 'what is wrong with me?' But 'what can I better understand about myself in relation to the society I live in and the experiences I have lived through?'

Scarves and safety

A weekly creative therapy group, made up of eight young men in a YOI, became a highly valuable space; this was a closed, time-limited group, offered to young people for 16 weeks at a time, with a new group beginning every four months. The connection between group members grew to be intuitive, honest and deeply rooted in shared experiences. Initially connection with peers on an emotional level was unfamiliar for most of the group members; this was apparent in the initial stages of group process, and, much like findings from Woodall's (2007) qualitative study, a significantly masculine ethos was created in the YOI environment and expressing difficulty was perceived as an act going against such masculine ideals. The groupwork provided the opportunity to facilitate exploration and 'challenge and reframe inherited traditional masculine ideals' (Lynch et.al 2018), whilst supporting the development of an internal framework for utilising the support of others, in a group setting, in a positive way that would not risk damage to perceived reputations (ibid). Within the YOI setting, reputation was held in high regard and was often the reason behind conflict and violent incidents.

The creation of an alternative physical environment was fundamental to enable group members to relate to each other in an alternative way than they had been within the prison environment. With regard to the room in which the therapy group took place, I reorganised the furniture to create a circle of chairs and a large table upon which I laid out various props, e.g. balls, scarves, bean bags and art materials. These objects immediately created cause for connection as group members laughed together about the nature of these items. 'Are we back in primary school?!' was something new group members noted over the years, immediately breaking the tension which was felt by all of us as we came together in an unknown space of a new group. I was initially concerned that I was infantilising these bright and considered young men and they hinted at such feelings. Mahmud once exclaimed to me in frustration, 'this is not what therapy is!' which led to a group discussion around if this is not therapy, then what is? Group members shared their understanding that it was somewhere to talk about your problems and somewhere that people who struggled with their mental health went to recover. It was suggested that in therapy a psychologist could interpret one's behaviour and let them know why they had been angry as a child or what had brought them to commit crime. Group members described expectations of an exposing, cold and clinical therapy environment; when asked about where relationship, trust and safety came into this, they boldly stated that they would never fully trust a professional.

Group members quickly began to make use of the tactile, colourful objects, which had initially been met with laughter and ridicule. These played an important part in the formation of the group and in emotional self-regulation; on entering the room, group members would pick up props, mainly balls, which they threw against the wall or squeezed and prodded, taking time to settle into the space and wait for all group members to arrive. These objects also played a part in building trust, such as in one session when a group member came in and immediately put a scarf over his head and face. The others laughed and then joined him. It is hard to describe the power in such a moment of group members mirroring each other's actions; each action has behind it a history of experience and in such a moment of mirroring, these two unique experiences meet. They joked about looking like women wearing wedding veils or headscarves. I remember a moment where tension crept up in my chest as I wondered cautiously what direction this would take; however, the group soon moved on from jokes and began to share news from their week. They told in-depth stories and appeared to listen carefully to each other. It felt easier for me to prompt them to reflect on their emotions and internal worlds; it appeared that risks were taken as trust was being developed. I wondered out loud at the positive impact of the scarves over faces, to which group members somewhat flippantly responded that yes, they did feel safer behind their scarves. As it had been imagery of women wearing scarves which had been conjured, it felt that in this masculine environment they needed to embody a sense of femininity to be able to metaphorically unveil more of themselves to me and their peers, whilst connecting with a more 'tender' culture of cooperation, sharing and nurture (Boas 2006: 119).

The scarves provided a sense of safety and cover, which had been absent in the descriptions of their imagined therapy environment. Here, the group had instinctively utilised the opportunity for innovation which this creative therapy environment offered, and they found a way to support themselves and each other to feel safer, and to ultimately begin the real work of the group.

Moving the power

Individual therapy sessions in the YOI environment would often take place in the small holding or meeting rooms behind the office on the prison wing. A large window adjoined the main office through which officers could see inside the room. It is worth mentioning here that clients could also look inside the office and often became distracted during sessions by the comings and goings of other prisoners and staff. The opportunity to be able to see what was going on for this small bit of time during which the clients were out of their cells was relished. Shaun, a client, once described the build-up of anxiety which he experienced whilst stuck in his cell for hours at a time, able to hear but not see what was happening on the wing. The sense of the power in information and knowledge was palpable. Shaun would come out of his cell for his session and constantly gather information from what he saw and heard around him. Being more in the know meant he could feel fractionally more in control.

Shaun, like many other care-experienced young people, came to therapy with the negative sense of his identity and with the sense that something was wrong with him. Care-experienced young people often find that social care and mental health services can pathologise their identities, and indirectly enhance negative feelings around them being 'bad, different or defective' (Colbridge et al. 2017: 12) when working within diagnostic systems which primarily focus on the 'deficits located within the individual' (ibid.12). Colbridge et al. (2017) noted that looked-after children and Care Leavers need intervention which is based on the goals of themselves, not the services around them, and that these interventions need to consider their strengths. They found that although much of Care Leavers' identities were formed through coping mechanisms and survival strategies, these were often seen as in need of treatment, with little consideration of the usefulness of these strategies in a young person's life. For care-experienced young people from Black, Asian and Minority Ethnic backgrounds, it is important to consider the numerous additional survival strategies which, as Thomas (1999) describes, develop from a young age to protect against prejudice and racism.

Shaun was a tall and broad young man who filled the room in which our session took place with his restless and anxious energy. He spoke rapidly, the words tumbling out of him one on top of the other. From the moment Shaun entered the room he would pace around it, often beginning with feelings of frustration as he spoke about the injustices he had experienced during the week, the fights he had been involved in and the punitive measures which he felt were vastly unfair. During our first session together, we heard a knock on the large window, following which a prison officer loudly reprimanded Shaun, saying 'you need to sit yourself down and engage'. This shaming intrusion was representative of the power dynamics of this youth offending establishment, reflecting the hierarchy where a uniformed officer felt able to interrupt a session held by a civilian member of staff. Shaun dipped his head and said to me: 'this is what I mean! They are always on me and it pisses me off!'

Shaun went on to tell me how persecuted he felt by people in positions of authority. As a civilian staff member, although I was not immediately put into the same category as the uniformed positions of authority to which he referred, as a therapist I came with an alternative association of power. An example of this came in a later session when Shaun told me that he was waiting to be judged and then diagnosed by me, evoking similar feelings he had experienced when standing up in court before a judge, waiting to be sentenced. As we explored what his expectation of therapy was, he shared that he thought we would have to sit on chairs across from each other and I would tell him what was wrong with him.

To facilitate trust and begin building a more mutual relationship, it was essential to address the power dynamic, to respond authentically and creatively to what Shaun was bringing, whilst vitally addressing the issue of body politics in such interactions with people in positions of power, working with the understanding that '…bodies are not neutral; gender, sexuality, ethnicity and class are socio-political aspects that shape our mental, emotional and physical selves and inform our ethical values' (Allegranti 2011: 487). It was important to create an environment with confidence, without a set of rules which excludes, but in which Shaun's own embodied process could be centred, thereby decolonising ideas of certain bodies holding importance and power and others not. We brought movement and embodied process to the forefront of our work and experimented with different ways to be present in the space, standing, shifting weight, pacing or creating patterns with our footsteps on the floor. Shaun would come up with ideas for us to try together, listening to what his physical self needed in the moment.

In the course of our work together, Shaun explored the strong feelings of failure which morphed into an overwhelming anger during his childhood when he was consistently told to learn to sit still and focus, to somehow contain the excess energy he had in his body, to still the racing thoughts in his mind. He shared his negative feelings towards teachers and carers who he felt had labelled him as 'naughty', 'disruptive', 'bad', 'angry' and then ultimately as he grew older, an 'aggressive and violent child'. He felt he had been consistently reprimanded for not being able to behave as others did, in the classroom or the home environment. Shaun tentatively began to make connections between his pent-up frustration and his violent outbursts, his school exclusions and the patterns of behaviour which had led to him being taken into care, moving between many placements, and encountering the criminal justice system, following which later he moved from a secure unit to a YOI.

Shaun's confidence in the responses he experienced in his body increased. Over time, he began to acknowledge that these were to be noticed and could be a strength which he could harness and that these bodily sensations could inform him of his emotions and of what was taking place internally. He became more conscious of the impact of the stress responses which flooded his body when recalling instances where he felt anger, frustration, disempowerment, humiliation and shame. In our work together, Shaun explored the painful events which triggered these emotions and the significance of his experiences in relation to those in positions of power and authority.

The initial stage of our embodied work enabled Shaun to feel empowered to take a lead in the therapy space in a way in which he had not expected. In experiencing a different power dynamic than he had previously, Shaun was able to begin to let go of some of the barriers which many young people report experiencing when accessing mental health support; these include the fear of judgement, of not being taken seriously or respected (Radez et al. 2021). The centring of movement and actively working with the presence of tension flow attributes of high intensity and bound flow, which Kestenberg-Amighi et al. (1999) suggest could reflect 'intensely felt anger, anxiety, pain or fear' (67), appeared to enable Shaun to begin to feel less judged and more attuned to (Erksine 1998; Stern 1985) in a way that had been missing from his early years and childhood, and which was currently absent in his experience in the prison environment.

Lynch et al. (2018) note that young men, in particular, wish to address their problems and seek support in an environment that provides some choice, control, and where there are equal power relations. Shaun's lived experience meant that he internalised a sense of both powerlessness and rage and struggled to acknowledge his strengths. Using movement, he was able to better integrate the emotional and physical aspects of himself (Payne 1992), to feel more in control and make active choices in his sessions. In working collaboratively with movement, the power was more shared. This enabled us to develop a trusting relationship in which we could work to understand more about his internal world, making links to how he responded to the society in which he lived. Fanon (Macey 2012) noted in his work to decolonise psychiatry and psychotherapy, that you cannot separate the imaginary life from the real world, that one must consider how the concrete world impacts the individual and adapt interventions according to the lived experience of the individual, in particular the context in which they experience the world. Shaun's sense of powerlessness was rooted in his lived experience of being brought up in systems excluded from the mainstream. By thinking creatively and bringing together these various aspects in the here and now therapy session, by enabling playfulness and an embodied therapeutic alliance, the therapy relationship was able to help Shaun to feel included and experience an empowerment that society had not frequently afforded him.

Dancing in the kitchen

Words hold a power which can create a barrier for young people accessing psychotherapeutic support. One client, Ciara, would tell me that her thoughts were going a 'million miles a minute' and moving so fast that it was hard to get a hold of the words, ultimately creating a feeling of being frozen.

Ciara and I spent many sessions sitting with the frozenness, feeling stuck together. We acknowledged the further challenge, when the words were finally grasped, to break through the barrier of fear of judgement, rejection and abandonment. It was easier to say nothing than to say something and risk this. I notice when writing this chapter, a parallel process of feeling stuck and paralysed with the fear of putting my words out there for others to judge.

As a society, we place so much importance on language and words. As professionals who are equipped with specific language through our training and study, we hold a sense of power which is absent from the experience of the young person who enters the therapy space. In some instances, clients are not yet equipped with words to describe their felt experience accurately and it may be that only sensations are present which are difficult to connect with emotional language. Perhaps trauma has occurred which is held primarily at a bodily level, or an emotional vocabulary simply has not been heard from others or learnt at any stage of their life, all leading to an overwhelming fear of saying the *wrong* words. Heyes et al. (2020) noted that another reported barrier to accessing support for young people was professionals using medicalised jargon. This was said to obstruct the formation of a safe and trusting relationship and some young people thought that some of the language used by professionals was confusing and unclear, and even sometimes cruel and dehumanising. Hast (2021) notes that language not only maintains hierarchies but also that '…language is not the only and most important form of knowledge.…if language is too abstract, to the point of being abstracted from experience, it is not accessible' (45). This applies to the therapy space on many levels and encourages me to reflect on the accessibility of not only the verbal language I use but my language as a Dance Movement Psychotherapist in my work with clients who do not always wish to actively create shape, form or rhythm in movement, but who are open to connecting on an embodied and sensory level.

In the initial stages of embedding a weekly creative therapy group in a setting with care-experienced young women, the group was set up to take place in the lounge area of a residential unit. The boundaries of the group were agreed such that the group would come together around a different creative activity, e.g. painting or crafting, which would be bookended by a verbal check-in and check-out, loosely echoing a Chacian structure (Chaklin & Schmais 1993) of a Dance Movement Psychotherapy group, but with the moving element taking place in the involvement with creative materials. The idea was to increase accessibility and make the space less threatening, the creative activity serving as a transitional object (Winnicott 1971) and bridging the space between us all. The introduction of the weekly group therapy space was met with some suspicion, the young women reflecting that they were not interested in therapy and expressing reluctance to share thoughts and feelings with each other and with a therapist who they did not know. The most involved group members at this time were young black women, who had varied interests, strengths and ambitions. The group made efforts to connect when I initially brought the suggestion of art-based creative activities, but it later transpired that for these group members this was not their first choice of activity through which to relate. Upon reflection I wonder if this process was on some level like what Thomas (1995) describes as *identification by proxy* whereby black and Asian children may go along with the narrative of the white professional, a strategy developed to protect themselves from a prejudiced society which has not always understood or welcomed their difference. I wonder if perhaps the initial acceptance of the art activities offered was akin to this. Although I am not a white worker and I am aware that my being a brown woman can at times positively impact the power dynamic. In instances like this, I can be viewed as white adjacent, in my position as a therapist which remains a predominantly white profession.

Before long, the group suggested we cook; it was put to me, 'if we can paint a picture why can't we cook a dish?' We came together in the kitchen, music was played in the background, with occasional bursts of singing along, bodies moved to the music and around each other, as things were rinsed, chopped and fried. It was a multi-sensory experience as the air was scented with cooking smells, warm with the heat of the oven and through the hands-on nature of food preparation, the sense of touch was alive. I was often looked to for guidance and advice, occupying a maternal role in the transference. Through my real-world errors, in providing the wrong ingredients; for example, on one occasion I was told that I had brought the utter worst brand of sweetcorn, I was frequently also the mother who was neglectful, uncaring and who got it wrong. In the here and now, I guided the group to reflect on the feelings which arose in these moments and in the process of problem solving, cooperation and compromise in the kitchen.

The way the group moved in space communicated a little more of everyone's personality. As a group we noticed, with sensitivity and non-judgement, the way we related to each other in the space: The speed and efficiency of one person, someone else who regularly got in people's way by trying to reach over or squeeze past, those who leant against the worktops and those who sat neatly in a chair. We noticed those who left a trail of crumbs behind them, and in contrast the person who cleaned and cleared up as we went. Almost imperceptibly we began to find times of mutual rhythm and a sense of co-regulation with each other, promoting a sense of safety and security. My kinaesthetic and sensory memory of what it was like to be in that space reminds me of the depth of connection on a non-verbal level.

This connection was only made possible by allowing the group to share power, to mutually navigate and co-create some of the more negotiable boundaries to shape the therapy space, forming an environment which offered the opportunity to connect on multi-sensory levels. It was only once the non-verbal, embodied connection had been established that thoughts, feelings and stories began to emerge. Prompted by the dissatisfaction in conflicting cooking methods, memories of mothers and grandmothers were spoken and what took place in the kitchens and homes of childhoods, the positive and negative experiences, were disclosed. The space was opened for a sharing of challenges and achievements of group members' daily lives. Importantly, the established environment gave the bodies in space the chance to continue to respond and regulate, the kitchen island was thumped in frustration, heads were occasionally thrown back in laughter, safety and regulation was sought in the subtle moments of someone turning away from the group towards the cold water tap when something was too painful. For this group to work, it had to be formed in this way and through this process, it meant that I had to centre the needs of the group and be open to create this space with them, as opposed to centring my need to offer my known and learnt way of running a group therapy space.

While I do not propose that group therapy always takes place in a kitchen, I advocate for working with adaptability and creativity to ensure that the therapy space is a warm and inviting place which can be cohabited for the duration of a session.

I attempt to demonstrate through these clinical vignettes that by creatively and imaginatively expanding the possibilities of what I could offer as a clinician, I was able to adjust my practice to the specific needs of my clients. I kept the question of what was useful for my clients at the forefront of my thinking and did this through consistently questioning, and at times struggling with the notion of how to challenge and reshape boundaries ethically, as I was striving to decolonise psychotherapeutic processes. Using creativity to enable a decolonising approach helped to address some of the barriers faced and by truly listening to client's subjective, intersectional, experience of living on the margins, their associations of clinical psychotherapy environments, and their experience of power and disempowerment, I put myself in the position of being the one to adapt creatively, rather than asking this of them. In a therapeutic relationship, we must acknowledge that the power relations will never be equal, and the therapist's role is to hold and contain the space. However, the act of naming this and providing a malleable environment which can be in some way co-created can go a long way in evening out the balance of power, whilst retaining containment, safety and the core of relational psychotherapeutic work.

References

Allegranti, B. (2011). Ethics and body politics: interdisciplinary possibilities for embodied psychotherapeutic practice and research. *British Journal of Guidance & Counselling*, 39 (5), pp. 487–500.

Alleyne, A. (2005). Invisible injuries and silent witnesses: the shadow of racial oppression in workplace contexts. *Psychodynamic Practice*, 11 (3), pp. 283–299.

Boas, S. (2006). The body of culture. In Payne, H. (ed.) *Dance movement therapy: theory, research practice*. Routledge, East Sussex, pp. 112–131.

Chaiklin, S. & Schmais, C. (1993). The Chace approach to dance therapy. In Sandel, S. L., Chaiklin, S. & Lohn, A. (eds.) *Foundations of dance movement therapy: the life and work of Marian Chace*. Maryland: The Marian Chace Memorial Fund, pp.

Colbridge, A. K., Hasset, A. & Sisley, E. (2017). *"Who am I?" how female care leavers construct and make sense of their identity*. Sage Open.

Crenshaw, K. (1989). Demarginalizing the intersection of race and sex: a black feminist critique of antidiscrimination doctrine. *Feminist theory and antiracist politics*, University of Chicago Legal Forum, 140, pp. 139–167.

Ellis, E. (2011). Towards a rainbow-coloured therapeutic community. *Psychotherapy and Politics International*, 9 (3), pp. 188–193.

Ellis, E. (2021). *The race conversation*. London: Confer books.

Erskine R. G. (1998). Psychotherapy in the USA: a manual of standardized techniques or a therapeutic relationship? *International Journal of Psychotherapy*, 3, pp. 231–234.

Hast, S. (2021). In touch with the mindful body: moving with women and girls at the Za'atari refugee camp. In Sepälä, T., Sarantou, M., & Miettinen, S. (eds.) *Arts-Based methods for decolonising participatory research*. New York: Routledge, pp.

Heyes, K., Craig, E., Gray, P., Whittenbury, K., Barclay, L., & Leigh, J. (2020). Young People and Mental health: How do young people want mental health support to be delivered? Youth and Policy https://www.youthandpolicy.org/articles/young-people-mental-health/.

HMPPS (2019). Care leavers in prison and probation. https://www.gov.uk/guidance/care-leavers-in-prison-and-probation.

Kestengerg-Amighi, J., Loman, S., Lewis, P. & Sossin, M. (1999). *The meaning of movement*. New York and London: Brunner-Routledge.

Lammy, D. (2017). The Lammy review. https://www.gov.uk/government/publications/lammy-review-final-report.

Lensvelt, I., Hasset, A., & Colbridge, A. (2021). More than meets the eye: how black and minority ethnic care-leavers construct and make sense of their identity. *Adolescents*, 1 (1), 3, pp. 6–53.

Lowe, F. (2014). Thinking space: the model. In Fakhry Davids, M. & Lowe, F. (eds.) *Thinking space: Promoting thinking about race, culture, and diversity in psychotherapy and beyond*. The Tavistock Clinic Series. London: Karnac, pp. 11–34.

Lynch, L., Long, M., & Moorhead, A. (2018). Young men, help-seeking, and mental health services: exploring barriers and solutions. *American Journal of Men's Health*, 12 (1), pp. 138–149.

Macey, D. (2012). *Frantz Fanon: a biography*. London: Verso Books.

Payne, H. (1992). Shut in, shut out. In Payne, H. (ed.) *Dance movement therapy: theory and practice*. London: Routledge, pp. 39–80.

Radez, J., Reardon, T., Creswell, C., Lawrence, P. J., Evdoka-Burton, G. & Waite, P. (2021). Why do children and adolescents (not) seek and access professional help for their mental health problems? A systematic review of quantitative and qualitative studies. *European Child & Adolescent Psychiatry*, 30, pp. 183–211.

Sanders, R. (2020). ESSS Outline: Care experienced children and young people's mental health. *Iriss*. https://doi.org/10.31583/esss.20201012.

Sepälä, T., Sarantou, M. & Miettinen, S. (2021). *Arts-based methods for decolonising participatory research*. New York: Routledge.

Stern, D. (1985). *The interpersonal world of the infant*. London: Basic Books.

Thomas, L. K. (1995). Psychotherapy in the context of race and culture: an intercultural therapeutic approach. In Fernando, S. (ed.) *Mental health in a multi-ethnic society*. London: Routledge, pp. 172–192.

Thomas, L. K. (1999). Communicating with a black child: overcoming obstacles of difference. In Milner, P. & Carolin, B. (eds.) *Time to listen to children*. London, Routledge, pp. 65–78.

Williams, D. R. (2018). Stress and the mental health of populations of color: advancing our understanding of race-related stressors. *Journal of Health and Social Behaviour*, 59 (4), pp. 466–485.

Winnicott, D. W. (1971). *Playing and reality*. London: Penguin.

Woodall, J. (2007). Barriers to positive mental health in a young offender's institution: a qualitative study. *Health Education Journal*, 66 (2), pp. 132–140.

Youth Access (2002). Breaking down the barriers: a strategy in development. www.youthaccess.org.uk.

Youth Justice Board (2015). Keeping children in care out of trouble: an independent review chaired by Lord Laming Response by the Youth Justice Board for England and Wales to the call for views and evidence. assets.publishing.service.gov.uk.

13 Sing your way home

Designing a creative group
intervention in the women's
prison as a Dance Movement
Therapist in Singapore

Agnes Law

The song we sang

Before I speak about the work, I want to tell you a personal story to highlight my motivation in writing this chapter. I come from a working-class family of Chinese and Malay ethnic origins in Singapore. Both of my grandmothers were born in China and Malaysia, respectively. As young girls, one was subjected to feet binding practice and the other was sold as a child slave. They were displaced from their families at a young age due to war. They experienced immense hardships from poverty to family violence. One developed mental health difficulties in her adulthood that resulted in her having to spend a long period of time away from her own children.

I was close to my paternal grandmother who was very prudent with her money. She knew the importance of education for girls, as she was not given one. She was adamant that her granddaughter should have an education and she paid for my school fees. She nicknamed me the 'female scholar' as I was the first female in my family to graduate with a degree and I know that she was proud of me. There is a Chinese saying 饮水思源 (yin shui si yuan), which literally translated means 'when one drinks water not to forget the source'. In other words, to urge younger generations to remember the labour of our ancestors. Because of the lived experience of my grandmothers, I felt strongly about providing a space for women's voices to be heard and to be empowered in my work.

My paternal grandmother sadly passed away in September 2020. Because of the travel restrictions due to the pandemic, I could not be by her side before she died. My memory goes back to when I was very young, when my grandmother would sing me a lullaby and rock me to sleep in a home-made hammock that hangs down from the ceiling. I was tucked safely in this hammock made out of a large coloured fabric joined by two safety pins and a metal spring together. This lullaby was the only song my grandmother had sung to me. I wondered if her own mother had sung the same song to her when she was young. Although I am not able to see my grandmother again, she has given me a song to remember her.

DOI: 10.4324/9781003222484-13

Sharing a song is a powerful gift you can give to someone when they are separate from their families and friends. This song, called *Sing Your Way Home*, became a popular song I have taught the women in the prison. To my knowledge, this is a children's song familiar to many who learnt it at school. Although I shared other songs with the women, this particular song stood out. Perhaps the lyrics of this song resonated with the women as they were missing their families. This song represents the unspoken wish the women had for one another as they anticipated their release from prison.

> *Sing your way home at the close of the day.*
> *Sing your way home; drive the shadows away.*
> *Smile every mile, for wherever you roam*
> *It will brighten your road, it will lighten your load*
> *If you sing your way home.*

(Verses from Sing your way home)

Introducing the creative project

The year after my graduation from Goldsmiths, University of London, I was working at a family centre in Singapore offering Dance Movement Therapy (DMT) in the community. When the invitation came to provide a bespoke programme for the women's prison, I agreed readily as I wanted to know how the knowledge I acquired in the United Kingdom could be adapted to a women's prison in Asia. In this project, other than DMT, I included additional creative resources in the group work that lean on my skills as a Playback Theatre practitioner.

The main features of the group work were dance, experiential and dramatising personal stories with the aims of building self-confidence and supporting the women's transition back to the community. Communications took place between colleagues from the family centre and the prison management to organise the logistics of the groupwork. With the help of two colleagues from the family centre, I facilitated several groups of pre-release women who received a total of 12 hours of psychological intervention over a four-week cycle. All names in this chapter have been changed to protect individual identities, and consent for writing about this work has been given by the relevant authority. For this creative project, I incorporated two creative disciplines in the group work which I am qualified to work in, namely DMT and Playback Theatre. DMT uses dance and movement to support the integration of body and mind within a psychological framework. Playback Theatre is a non-scripted and improvised drama based on the personal stories of participants. In this chapter, I will discuss the question in practice; that is, how does the group facilitator support women to feel safe, to attune to their body and to express themselves in a time limited therapeutic group? I will use observations, reflections and a description of the group process to illustrate the themes of the work.

Prior to designing the group work, I was given basic information about the women: name, age, index offence and release date. They were of different ethnic backgrounds and their ages ranged from late teens to late fifties. Most of them were in prison for drug related offences and a few had offended previously. The women were selected by the prison management and grouped according to their release dates. Unlike other work I had carried out in a family centre, this was a unique experience stepping into the women's prison and offering a psychological intervention rooted in arts, therapy and theatrical expression. After communications with the prison management, I brought in my own props for the group work, which consisted of cloths, music and art materials. I imagined feeling lost without my props as these were 'barang saya' (from Malay language translate 'my things') which formed part of my professional identity. I can see now that my 'barang' provided an ice-breaker in my initial encounters with the women.

Establishing a sense of safety and self-care in the group context

I began the group with some apprehension as to how much I could offer with such a time limited intervention. Safety came to mind and I adapted my understanding of group therapy by introducing the therapeutic principles of boundaries and consistency in the sessions. I demarcated the beginning and the ending of the session with a predictable structure. I was given only basic information about the women and no way to find out about their relationship with each other in the prison. In hindsight, an assessment with the women would have been useful to learn about their needs before matching them in their groups. As my contact with each group of women was limited, I had to find a therapeutic stance that I felt comfortable to take on, which included emotional holding and containment for the participants. Hence, I started with asking the women to share their hopes and fears they might have in attending such a group together.

I then introduced a group contract and discussed expectations and goal setting with the women. I explained to the group that being an external facilitator who only has access to the prison while running these sessions, I would like to hear how they were coping in the prison. I emphasised that the group space belonged to the group and it was designed to be a safe and confidential space. However, I added a safeguarding clause that I would pass on information to the management if they disclosed plans to hurt themselves or others. I explained that confidentiality meant our conversations would stay in the group space and urged them not to share with others when they returned to their cells. I observed the responses of the women were rather quiet and they were probably unsure of how to use this group space at the beginning.

Part of the group work was about supporting the women to develop self-awareness and metaphorically to sing their way back to the source of their creativity. I wanted to introduce creativity and movement at the beginning.

Psychoanalyst, Winnicott (1971) spoke about the importance of play and creativity which supports the understanding of self (63). I introduced games to get the women moving and build cooperation. These dramatic games such as Charlie's Angel, Zip Zap Zop and Earthquake (Fox 2010) served as ice-breakers for the group. The group's alliance began to form as we became immersed in the participation of these games. These energisers were fun and eased the women's anxieties of participation. Self-disclosure circle was a useful activity to build rapport as we began to find out about each other's likes and dislikes in the group.

Language was an important factor contributing to the safety of the group. Given the diversity of the participants, other than English, I included the use of the women's preferred languages (Mandarin Putonghua and Bahasa Malay) in the sessions. My two colleagues provided invaluable support in building the group's trust. I carried out the group facilitation in English, and my colleagues provided the translation as and when required. Whenever possible, I would group the participants into their preferred language to have smaller group conversations facilitated by each of my colleagues. I watched the participants become animated in their bodies as they spoke in their native languages, which perhaps was a way of them connecting back to their own ancestral source. As each session progressed, I observed them gaining more confidence relating to us.

While I was carrying out this work, I sought supervision from an experienced DMT supervisor to reflect on my experiences as a group facilitator. Not wanting to infantilise the participants, I needed to reflect on my unconscious bias. I held compassion for the women and at the same time, I worried about the challenges that awaited them in the society after their release. I reflected on the complexity of emotions and the transference I picked up from the therapeutic work. My colleagues and I were in touch with feelings of sadness and anger in our debriefing. There seemed to be a parallel process that was happening as I was feeling disempowered in my professional work life; unbearable feelings were at play in the transference and countertransference. I was also carrying feelings of 'impotence' in my role and oscillating between 'feeling stuck' and 'feeling mobilised'. In hindsight, I recognised these were countertransference responses we picked up from the therapeutic work and I now wish there was adequate supervision offered to us while we were working on this project. In the absence of group supervision, it was important our team was able to find other ways of self-care and support through spirituality, meditations and shared values in order not to lose sight of our collective vision to support these women.

Building connections through dance and movements

Prior to working in the prison, I did not know how the participants of Asian backgrounds would respond to dance experiential work. The word 'dance' brought up some confusion for them. I observed their initial reactions as if

I could read their minds 'are we allowed to dance in the prison?' or 'I am not a dancer' and 'I don't know how to move'. I adopted a Chacian structure (Levy 2015) for the dance experiential and I took the opportunity to address their reservations by reassuring them during the verbal check in. I stressed the dance experiential was not a performance and no one would be judged on their dance. As a DMT, I was constantly attuning to the many different cues from the women to get some feedback on the group process. Siegel (1984) spoke about observing the entire person, including their posture, breathing, tone and the rhythm of their voice to give you an indication of their needs. She suggested that theme arises when one engages in the dance.

At the start of the dance experiential, I introduced breathing exercises to support their physical grounding. I used visualisation before warming up the body parts such as stretching arms and limbs outwardly in different directions. The facilitated warm up then developed into a mirroring activity of a movement and a gesture, rotating the leadership in the group where each participant took turn to lead in the dance improvisation. The warm up exercises and dance were accompanied by contemporary pacific music soundtrack (Vaka 1997). The musical choice was a deliberate one to support the women to freely associate their movements with the music unfamiliar to them. This type of percussion music provided the impetus in the group for the women to dance together. The role of mirroring supported the development of empathy and the sense of connection within the group. After the dance experiential, we sat down and reflected on our experience. The women generally enjoyed moving with one another. Some experienced an instant relief from the pre-occupations they had arrived with, as they reported physical pains (headache or stomach pain) dissipating after the dance. I was convinced that the women found a physical release in their body from the dance experiential. Moving supported the regulation of their feelings and enhanced their somatic awareness. Below is a vignette to illustrate a group participant's experience:

> As soon as the music began, the smiles appeared on their faces. Each participant took a turn to lead and follow one another. Their bodies began to soften as they moved into the space around the room. They were offering eye contact, offering open gestures and mirroring back to one another. They swayed to the rhythms and waved their hands holding bright and colourful fabrics, and some even dressed up in them. The atmosphere seemed light and joyful. Afterwards, Aysha shared this: 'In here, the officer calls me by the number[1] on my attire, but after dancing, I remember who I am. My name is Aysha'. Aysha went on to say 'I feel free when I dance, I am relaxed and I do not have the headache anymore'.

During the dance experientials, props such as scarfs, cloths of different colours and textures were available to provide the group the opportunities to move with a prop and to form connections with others. The props seemed to be a favourite among the women as they found themselves dressing up with the cloths. After the dance, the women often spoke about the contrast of their dancing when they were moving with these coloured cloths, having forgotten momentarily that they were wearing prison attire. Using scarves or coloured cloths gave the women permission to show off their personality in the dance. The women explored different ways to dress themselves up; wearing a headscarf or as a skirt or dancing along with the cloth. They were twirling, flicking, folding or following their body impulses spontaneously dancing with others.

I observed the marked difference in the women's bodies as they moved confidently along the sagittal plane, advancing and retreating within the group space, sometimes as if we were on the runway show. Different people took 'the spotlight' to show off their new outfit and sashayed to the music while the rest of the group cheered on like supportive fans. It was moving to witness the women in this 'dress up dance', and to see the exhilaration and the joy on their faces as they swayed along with the music. Now reflecting back, I connect to the theme of loss of personal identity these women experienced within the institution. Perhaps dancing with the colourful fabrics helped the women to reclaim their femininity.

For this creative programme, I wanted to encourage the use of spontaneity in their body in order to increase personal awareness. For instance, apart from the dance experientials, I facilitated structured activities to move in pairs, borrowing ideas from Anne Bogart's viewpoints and effort theories from Laban Movement Analysis. I demonstrated some of the movement postures, for instance, exploring how to move in relation to another person. We worked with still images or sculptures, and we also moved our body in different directions and levels. I would get the women to move in pairs to show oppositional movement such as strong and light weight or free and bound flow from Laban's effort theory (Newlove & Dalby 2004). I sometimes added in the challenge of allowing the pairs to pick a few of their movement signatures and to perform in front of the group. Some spoke about developing confidence in sharing their movement and having fun in the process. Reflecting back, perhaps I could have provided more time to allow the quieter members of the group to speak in order to gauge how they were integrating their experiences in the group.

Deepening group awareness with personal stories told in action

One of the aims of the group was to support the women's transition as part of their release. I asked them to share their thoughts and feelings as they approached their release date. Some were open in their sharing and spoke about mixed feelings of excitement to see their children and families, but also of nervousness about securing work as an ex-offender. I could see they were troubled by this anticipated transition. With the earlier cohorts, I provided some skills training for the women such as setting goals before their

Agnes book!

Please borrow if
you would like
to read — but
bring back!

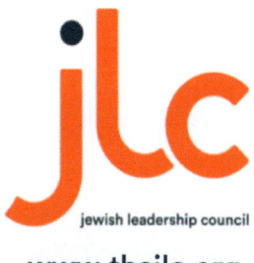
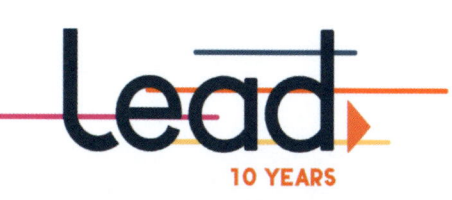

release. On reflection, I felt there were stories waiting to be told based on the drawings the women created during our reflection time together. Hence, I wanted to provide a space for deeper conversations to take place. I introduced a timeline activity to encourage the women to share significant events that happened in their lives. Some chose to speak about the offence, and some went on to reminisce about their childhood.

Back to the mission of empowering the women to tell their stories, I introduced a drama element in the group work. I am a practitioner of Playback Theatre which is a form of improvised theatre based on personal stories. Playback Theatre is practised across the world and as a theatre form it has its own traces in education, community and commercial sectors. Rowe (2007) stated that Playback provides the opportunity for silent stories to be told and he argues for Playback Theatre to be seen as a social intervention. I believe in the power of Playback Theatre to provide the vehicle of transformation in my community. Jonathan Fox, the co-founder of Playback Theatre, writes about the use of 'citizen actor' in Playback Theatre (Rowe 2007) that the people can perform as needed. For the women's group work, I acted as a Playback Theatre conductor inviting stories to be told and providing a framework that considers the relationship between art, social interaction and Playback rituals (Fox & Dauber 1999). Playback Theatre was a way of encouraging empathic connections between the group participants.

Unlike in a Playback Theatre performance where I would have an ensemble of trained Playback actors to act out the stories, I had to devise a way which would work in the context of the group. Working in small groups, after the timeline activity, I asked the women to choose one of the personal stories shared. Then, they asked the teller permission to act out their story. They rehearsed the story and worked in partnership for the role play. They could use movement gestures, dialogue and props, such as cloths, to act out the rehearsed story in front of others. More commonly, the personal stories acted out were domestic in nature such as cooking, eating, talking and going out together. A few acted out the reasons that got them arrested; for instance, they were caught glue sniffing at a friend's place. It could be argued that the sharing of personal stories might be triggering for some. Therefore, the role of the facilitator is important as they play a vital role in observing and naming the emotional experiences that are unfolding in the group.

After the role playing, I introduced the Playback stage (Salas 2001) and invited my colleagues and the women to volunteer the acting for the whole group. I prepared the volunteer actors that there would be no discussion on how to act out the stories, as is the case with Playback Theatre performance where the aim is spontaneity in action. As a conductor, I asked the women to offer feelings associated with their group experience so far and these were enacted with sounds and movements by the volunteer actors. I proceeded by asking if any women wished to tell a personal story in the witness of the whole group. After each enactment, I acknowledged the teller and asked for their response in seeing their story being acted out. The cycle of eliciting stories in Playback (Chesner & Hanh 2002) creates a collage of themes present in the group. I was reminded of stories from childhood as themes of winning and losing, and the hopes about the future were shared. After the Playback experience, I found that the women started to relate on the themes and their connections with one another went deeper.

From the group conversations with the women, we discovered that there were mothers missing their children who were being cared for by families. Although this was by no means a representation of this client population, some common themes seemed to emerge from their childhood stories such as deprivation and emotional neglect. After the Playback Theatre experience, I suggested that the women pen or draw their feelings or thoughts in their journal. Journaling became a way of containing their group experience. Sometimes, I chose a lyrical type of music to play in the background while the women were journaling. Towards the end of the year with the later cohorts of women, I noticed I became confident with less content in the group structure and allowing more supportive conversations to take place in the sessions.

The effect of telling one's stories on a Playback Theatre platform can be profound as the teller becomes their own catalyst of transformation. Although I was not able to check in with the tellers after the group had ended, I could only draw on my own experience of doing Playback Theatre that the experience of sharing one's story stays with the teller for a long time. The employment of active listening skills and empathy using Playback Theatre can bring about immense benefits for the women, one of which being empowering these women to come forward to tell their stories and to reconnect with the source of their own historical waters. I feel strongly that this process of asking stories in Playback Theatre brings out a parallel dynamic that mirrors the group's lived experiences, which relates to their sense of belonging, validation and self-worth.

Conclusion

This creative project is my attempt in using a transdisciplinary approach combining DMT, Playback Theatre and singing to create a facilitating environment for these women in the prison. Clarity of the group structure and working with translations encouraged participation from the women at the outset. The facilitator referred to psychological theories, such as the psychodynamic model, to develop understanding of unconscious communications in the group dynamics. DMT group skills were used to support the emotional holding of the women in the group. The themes of loss, hope and belonging weaved through the sessions like a red thread from the beginning to the end of the groupwork.

The group facilitator's use of shared leadership and mirroring contained feelings of anxiety around participation. Learning through action opened a space for the women to find their own voice and to share their personal stories. Spontaneity was the key to creativity as the women immersed themselves in the play and enactment of stories afterwards. Dance and movement supported the women to release stress located in their body and free up thinking space to manage troubling thoughts. The experiential nature of the group activity promoted self-expression and increased self-awareness. Singing increased engagement in the women and at the same time provided a space for group participants to find belonging. Porges (2011) stated the benefits of singing and vocalisation for our human body and emotional resilience. The activity of singing together increased the feeling of safety for the women, regulated their physiological responses and supported their participation in the group. The group's singing experience provided a contrast to the other group activities. Singing is inclusive, allowing all to participate at the same time and it bonds the group together.

In this chapter, I have explored the weaving of different creative approaches adapted from DMT and Playback Theatre for a group of female prisoners in Southeast Asia. In recalling my work with this group of women, I have considered how creating and telling our story, past, present and future, is a process of emancipation and growth.

Note

1 The organisation is no longer using this practice (calling prisoners by their number).

References

Chesner, A. & Hahn, H. (2002). *Creative advances in group work*. London: Jessica Kingsley Publishers.

Fox, H. (2010). *Zoomy Zoomy: Improv games and exercises for groups*. New York: Tusitala Publishing.

Fox, J. & Dauber, H. (1999). *Gathering voices: Essay on playback theatre*. New York: Tusitala Publishing.

Levy, F. (2015). *Dance movement therapy: A healing art*. Reston: America Alliance for Health.

Newlove, J. & Dalby, J. (2004). *Laban for all*. New York/London: Routledge.

Porges, S. (2011). *The polyvagal theory: Neurophysiological foundations of emotions, attachment, communication, and self- regulation*. London: W.W. Norton & Company.

Rowe, N. (2007). *Playing the other: Dramatizing personal narratives in playback theatre*. Great Britain: London/Philadelphia: Jessica Kingsley Publishers.

Salas, J. (2001). *Improvising with real life: Personal story in playback theatre*. New York: Tusitala Publishing.

Siegel, E.V. (1984). *Dance movement therapy: Mirror of ourselves. The psychoanalytic approach*. New York: Human Sciences Press.

Vaka, T. (1997). *Te Vaka original contemporary pacific (Warm earth records)*. Auckland: Spirit of Play Productions Ltd.

Winnicott, D.W. (1971). *Playing and reality*. London: Tavistock Publications.

14 Borderlands

Exploring creativity as a practice of liminality in the arts therapies

Marina Rova and Marrianne Behm

Introduction

Dialogic meaning making is at the heart of this piece of writing. The text is shaped by different voices and creative explorations. We, Marrianne and Marina, write as therapists, artists, colleagues, women, migrants, mothers and researchers. Our writing is informed by the stories of four women with whom we worked as part of a mixed-modality arts therapies group within an adult outpatient mental health service (National Health Service UK). We also build on the voices of other authors, scholars, artists and practitioners who inspire and nourish our practice and writing. As such, this chapter presents a constellation of multiple perspectives and understandings of creativity as a practice of liminality in psychotherapeutic work.

We had been passing this book chapter back and forth between us, responding to each other's words, reviewing archives, old notes and images. Meeting on Zoom, we engaged in lively discussion as we recalled significant moments in the group. We were looking back to a process more than two years after it was completed. In our latest conversation, we asked each other to share what we were in touch with as we reflect on the process of revisiting the material.

MARRIANNE: 'It is where we met…'
MARINA: 'Yes, the things that connected…'
MARRIANNE: 'The separateness that wouldn't exist without the connection!'
MARINA: 'That's right, connection clarified our differences and togetherness at the same time.'
MARRIANNE: 'And this happened over time…'
MARINA: 'Giving space for something to evolve….I am struck by the personal resonance I feel reconnecting with the work, as a woman and an immigrant but also as a mother etc.'
MARRIANNE: 'Yes, there was a shared experience of "outsideness"… but also the risks we took as therapists in trusting each other in the space…'

This chapter explores creativity as a practice of liminality drawing from our collaboration as co-facilitators in a cross-modal dance movement and art

DOI: 10.4324/9781003222484-14

psychotherapy group for women living with depression. Cross-modal work is a developing clinical approach in the arts psychotherapies (Burrell & Cohen 2018; Colbert & Bent 2018; Rova et al. 2020). We argue that the creative process, cultivated through both embodied and visual approaches, can hold liminal experiences safely and meaningfully.

Central to this chapter is the idea of the client/therapist's motif taking a transformative journey as it moves across art forms. We shall explore how the richness and variety of the journey across modalities creates a space for reflection and a way to reconnect with ourselves. We shall also consider creativity as a space for possibilities and how the threshold of liminality can act as a container for potential and change. Furthermore, by integrating the different art forms, new boundaries are established, for example between moving, art making and verbalising, which the therapist and client need to jointly negotiate. In other words, the traditional hierarchical power of the therapist and client is suspended as both step into the liminal space. This shared experience can help clients gain a stronger sense of the boundary between the self and others and hence their own identity.

The process of writing this chapter illuminates to us how we are doing so from within another liminal space as we consider the group from the post-Brexit, pandemic-stricken reality of 2021. Isolation, loneliness, separation, alienation, loss and displacement are words that many people can relate to during troubling times. For the four women in our group however, these well-trodden narrative paths extend all the way to early childhood trauma. The grip of depression can be debilitating. It often breeds insecurity and indecisiveness. Group participation involved a lot of effort and perseverance from both sides: the clients prioritising and committing to the work and the therapists ensuring that contact was not lost, especially after absences or when resistance (to engage in the work) was palpable. And yet, over time, we identified a number of factors that gave the women resources, enhanced their agency and provided them with a safe space to experience themselves differently. These included the repetitive nature of the therapeutic process, the known movement props and art materials, the physical and emotional containment of the therapy room, the familiar faces around the circle, the shared stories and collective memories cultivated, the playful potentiality of the creative process and the group rituals and conventions. We started each session from a place of 'not knowing' and ended with more clarity, not certainty. The implicit (knowing), always there but out of sight, became explicit (known), seen and witnessed.

Claxton (2015) states that '(w)e exist by happening' (36). This 'happening' occurs time and again, from womb to birth to each developmental phase, rite of passage and transition that we encounter throughout the lifespan. Anyone who has experienced the arduous and (often) painful process of therapy work will recognise these rites of passage in their personal story and growth. Creativity, the act of *being-in-the-making* to paraphrase Grayson Perry (2021) is arguably not only our innate (human) capacity but also what brings us closest to the (animate and inanimate) world that we inhabit. We, the authors, consider creativity as embodied, processual, situated, contextual and relational. Poet and musician Kae Tempest (2020) writes '(c)reativity is the ability to feel wonder and the desire to respond to what we find startling. Or, more simply, creativity is any act of love' (5). This sense of wonder Tempest describes can be seen vividly in the imaginative play of children. Like play, creative processes open up liminal spaces of possibility and multiplicity. It is this space (and place) in-between that we describe as *borderlands* and that we will dwell in, in this chapter. In other words, to enter into play is to transition into a different state of being, a liminal state:

> Start by ridding yourself of the idea that play is subjective and egocentric. It is actually the opposite. Play requires immersion in "otherness". I get out of myself when I play and I enter an imaginative realm that is a distinctly different state of being.
>
> McNiff (1998: 117)

Van Gennep (1960) conceptualised liminality (from the Latin limen for threshold) as the place in between a neither-here-nor-there transitional state of being. What liminality then articulates in praxis is a process of transformation, a metamorphosis. Through the clinical examples we discuss, we will suggest that embodied creative practice is, in and of itself, a valid inquiry into lived experience. We value creative psychotherapeutic work as an important approach to both knowing and *knowledging*. The meaning or stories we create are constantly shaped by others and our environment. Practice-based approaches allow for direct access to this experiential (lived) knowing. Furthermore, we will illustrate that the creative process opens up a multidimensional sensorial space for making sense of our experiences in the world.

We begin with an overview of the context of the therapeutic work we explore in this chapter. We then *enter* the borderlands as we recall three vignettes from the creative process revealing moments of liminality and transformation. To protect the confidentiality of the group members, the vignettes we share in this chapter have been altered and pseudonyms are being used throughout. Finally, we conclude by considering creativity as an enhancer of reflexivity and integration; a process of becoming (who we are), and thus finding our way back home.

The mixed-modality group

The service within which the group took place was established by Marrianne, an art psychotherapist by training, in 1997. Marina joined the arts therapies team, as a dance movement psychotherapist, in 2010. We had been working with mixed modalities in the Arts Psychotherapies Department for many years, with different art forms being offered in the same session (Behm 2022; Burrell & Cohen 2018). For this group, we wanted to go one stage further and explore the liminal space or border between the art forms. In other words, we wanted to give clients, not just an experience of different arts modalities, but an immersion in a continuous creative process, which passes through modalities. As psychotherapists we had both experienced, on a personal level, the way in which a liminal space between art forms can be transformative and we wanted to explore whether this was something that would benefit our clients.

Arts psychotherapy groups vary considerably in the amount of structure they use. For example, some groups leave art making materials for the group to engage with when the need arises and other groups have a regular set structure. In planning this group, it occurred to us that a regular structure was needed to provide our client group, of women with severe depression and trauma, with a sense of safety. Furthermore, given the levels of low motivation with which we were faced, we felt that, as therapists, we should model engagement in the arts for the group members. This also enabled us to suspend the traditional hierarchical client-therapist dynamic and an opportunity for play opened up as we all stepped into the liminal space. Dismantling hierarchical power dynamics was not without its challenges, however, as we continued to hold clinical responsibility for the work. One participant consistently reminded us of the power-laden dynamics of our position in the group by calling us 'Head Marrianne and Doctor Marina'. As co-facilitators, we also had to navigate our own relational dynamics, including stepping in and out of the leader position as we took turns to facilitate the creative process. We felt that a structured group would enable us to participate, whilst also holding the boundaries to ensure the group remained a safe space. The structure also held the potential for both free flowing, spontaneous, improvisation and guided creative process to unfold. The group process unfolded over three cycles of 12 sessions each. Each session lasted for one hour and fifteen minutes. An evaluation process, at the beginning and end of the therapeutic programme, supported clients to monitor their progress.

The session started with members checking in with the group by choosing a card (from a selection of images) or object to represent how they felt in the present. This ritual was repeated each week and had the effect of including members as participants in the group and of engaging them in symbolising how they felt. This bridging of felt sense with symbolic articulation during the check-in offered a supportive way into the process for this group of women, all of whom had English as a second language. The next section focused on bringing awareness to our moving bodies. This developed into solo, partner or group movement improvisation which led into the art making process. Participants mostly worked on their own images sharing a large table and a range of dry and paint materials. The penultimate phase of the session involved group reflection with reference to the created art work (displayed upon a large table), the shared movement experiences and relational dynamics in the group. The session ended with a final grounding or centring exercise and a (verbal or non-verbal) check out.

As can be seen, our structure alternated embodied expression with expression through visual media and was aimed at disrupting the boundary between the two to enable clients to move their motif across art forms. Whilst our modalities, of art psychotherapy and Dance Movement Psychotherapy are distinct professional and clinical disciplines, we consider them both to be embodied and visual as creative and therapeutic practices. To this end, we use the term motif to denote the formulation or crystallisation of creative and therapeutic patterns observed across the modalities. This use of structure to disrupt is akin to anthropologist Turner's (2017) conceptualisation of the liminal space. Turner developed Van Gennep's idea of liminality as a transitional and transformational space occurring with rites of passage, where the structure of the ritual is used to disrupt existing symbols and structures to create something new.

The fact that we, as therapists, participated in the creative process heightened the sense of immersion in each stage of our structured group. It also meant we could follow the transition from one art form to another and respond to what group members were exploring in using the same medium, for example, mirroring a movement or creating an image in response to the other images. We also found that cross-modal references appeared in the creative process organically, for example in visual metaphors illustrated through the movement and through embodied qualities observed in the art making. For example, the large stretch cloth used during the movement improvisation conjured up an image of a wave. Similarly, embodied effort qualities punctuated the art making process as different art materials animated the women's bodies differently. Imagine the striking juxtaposition between a delicate and barely visible pencil trace and the indulgent sploshing of oil paint on a large piece of paper. This non-verbal dialogue within artistic practice has similarities with the non-verbal parent–infant interaction observed by Winnicott (1971), who described this relational space as an intermediate area of experience. Winnicott conceived of the play between infant and carer as a transitional space and we could compare this space to a liminal space. Trevarthen (1983) described the parent–infant interaction as involving a fusion of musical intonation and dance and is therefore very much a play between the art forms. This sense of play allowed clients to explore their fixed positions and take their motifs on a transformational journey.

Stories from the borderlands

'The man feels lonely'

Sandra, who lived with severe depression and trauma, began the first part of the session by choosing a card of a thick set heavy looking man standing alone against a backdrop of a flat landscape and a horizon. The man was looking away with his back turned to the viewer. In the movement part of the session, she explored weighted qualities through a series of strong and light movements. This evolved into her playing with transferring her weight by leaning back into thick elastic bands held by the therapists and group members, who supported her weight and then allowed her to spring back into an upright position. In the art making section of the group, she returned to the theme present in her card: a person alone against a flat landscape. However, she painted herself in the place of the man and changed the position so she was looking forwards towards the viewer. Notably, when she chose the card of the man, Sandra described feelings of loneliness in the third person: 'the man feels lonely'.

Sandra talked about the man in the image being lonely as if to say, 'this is not about me'. Sandra struggled to connect to her feelings and this form of dissociation is often observed in people experiencing depression. When she stepped into the movement space, Sandra connected to her weight, and therefore found her felt sense. The elastic band pressed against her body as she yielded into this physical boundary. When she created her artwork, she replaced the man in the image with herself. Not only that, she chose to turn towards the viewer, allowing herself to be seen. We could suggest that Sandra painted herself, allowing herself to be seen by her perceived viewer who, in this context, was no other than herself. Through this process of becoming, Sandra revealed herself to herself.

This substitution in the image, and thus Sandra's shift into an embodied (first-person) position supported her to articulate feelings of loneliness that she also linked to the loss of her role as a mother and a wife. She talked about her feeling of heaviness, something that the group had also experienced in relation to her as well as noticing the flatness in her voice. We might see the idea of weight as being central to a motif that was transformed through a journey between art forms. Reflecting on her painting, she made a link back to the earlier movement work where she felt supported by the group for the first time. This act of supporting her weight appears to have helped transform her sense of heaviness. The changes between the image and the card are small but significant. Like the man in the post card, she stands alone, a solid figure against a flat landscape but unlike the man she faces the viewer, her body is upright and open. We might see this as symbolic of her feeling for the first time supported by the group and able to face the group and disclose her feelings. This change occurred in the movement work but was articulated more fully in her art making. We might also see her art making as a synthesis of movement work and image making, because she is physically embodied at the centre of a visual image. Visual images enable a sense of perspective. In choosing the card, Sandra gained a safe distance from the immediacy of her process. However, in engaging with her material creatively something was set in motion, which subsequent movement work and art making brought together so that she became the centre of her image.

'The eagle'

Rose, who also experienced severe depression, chose a card with an image of an eagle. Notably, she chose the card just before the therapist could get to it, in a kind of swooping movement. Initially, there was not an obvious connection between the client, who was physically frail, and the eagle image and, like the example above, she did not say she identified with the image. However, in the movement section, unprompted, she found herself making movements that seemed like flight and explored flying as the eagle. In the art making section, the swooping swirling motions transformed into a forest waterfall and she reflected on feeling a sense of power. We might see this as a journey that started with a challenge to the therapist over a card that then moved into the development and embodiment of an image of a powerful bird of prey.

Whereas in the previous example Sandra's connection to the initial image could be described as concrete in the literal and symbolic sense of the word, here the resonance Rose has with this wild bird of prey is transformational. Rose's choice of image is both bold and playful. Most importantly, it allows her to articulate invisible parts of herself to the group. Rose, as the eldest and frailest member of the group, did not embody the eagle's agility in a literal sense, though she enjoyed exploring bird movements as part of the creative process. However, it was her quick wit and often challenging views that echoed the eagle's temperament, thus highlighting her powerful influence in the group.

'Red and black'

In the example above, the group member found a way to embody the image she chose. However, at other times the transition between the image and the body was less straightforward. For example, Valeria, who also lived with severe depression and medically unexplained pain symptoms, began the session by choosing a red and black image of intestines, which she said reminded her of a medical scan she was due to have. At this point, her connection with the image was largely factual. During the body awareness section, she described having a sensation of a large heavy mass inside her. Movement work allowed her to play with this sensation and she felt she was able to jiggle the mass around a little. During the art making section, she painted a large black rock, which appeared to connect with the hard heavy mass she explored during the movement section. She then added red and transformed the image into a red and black volcano. During the group discussion, she reflected that the volcano represented her buried anger. In this example, it is notable that the hard heavy mass expressed in the movement work was not really a straightforward embodiment of the card of the red and black intestines. Indeed, the connection to the intestines was only really apparent in the final volcano image, which used the same red and black colour scheme but also incorporated the hard rock like mass present in the movement work.

In this example, body sensations and imagery are more fragmented and only take a coherent integrated form at the end. At this point the client is also able to symbolise by seeing the volcano as an articulation of her buried anger. We can relate this journey towards symbolisation to developmental stages. Initially, the infant is aware of fragmented body sensations; during the mirror stage, the infant develops an image of its own body and then later internal images are symbolised through a shared system of communication (Bailly 2009). To some extent, Valeria re-traced this developmental process. Her initial image of intestines was not symbolised and was simply connected to the fact of her appointment to look into her unexplained symptoms of pain. Difficulties in symbolising are often present in people, who have medically unexplained symptoms where the symptom is a somatisation of psychological pain. The body awareness section connected the group member to fragmented sensations of heaviness and hardness. However, movement work enabled these to form an image or a hard mass. The art-work further articulated this image until it became something recognisable to the client and she was able to see it as a symbolic manifestation of her anger.

Closing reflections

We have described the work of a mixed-modality arts psychotherapy group that was structured as a series of stages. As we have discussed, this structure was repeated each week like a ritual, creating a sense of familiarity and safety within which risks could be taken. For example, as the weeks progressed, the group became more comfortable and relaxed with the opening ritual of choosing a card or object and Rose, who had spent many weeks waiting for others to choose cards, finally took a risk and swooped in on the card she wanted ahead of the therapist. Notably at this point, Rose did not know what the eagle represented but was open to exploring it further. This willingness to take a risk or a chance and embark on a journey into the unknown was a feature of our group as '(t)he creative process blends structure with chance' (McNiff 1998: 18).

A psychologist's article in *The New York Times* became viral during the pandemic, as it was shared millions of times on social media. Grant (2021) discusses languishing as the in-between phase between depression and flourishing, where passivity, lack of focus and an overall absence of well-being may be present. 'Languishing is a sense of stagnation and emptiness. It feels as if you're muddling through your days, looking at your life through a foggy windshield' Grant (2021) explains (available online at https://www.nytimes.com/2021/04/19/well/mind/covid-mental-health-languishing.html).

Flow is considered to be the antidote for languishing which can be achieved through uninterrupted time engaging with a simple task. Immersing ourselves in the creative process goes a step further. It opens up our experiential receptivity, it connects us to our senses, our animal body, our imagination and felt sense and it allows us to inhabit our home-of-beingness more meaningfully. We observed flow in the work of these women as they transitioned from one experiential process to the next, as they became more animated and as they connected to their vitality (Stern 2010).

As can be seen from the vignettes explored in this chapter, group members often achieved clarity at the end of the process. Before this point, they went through transitional or liminal states, which helped articulate their motif into something that could be named and related to themselves. Central to this process was the movement between modalities which broke up our standard cultural conceptions of dance and art as very separate modalities. The mixed-modality approach supported group members to explore image making and embodiment differently to how they would in a single-modality approach. Mixing the two together gave group members a strong sense of stepping in and out of their perceived reality. This facilitated the formation of an image that felt connected to self both symbolically and physically. The microcosm of the liminal space of the group echoed the bigger life thresholds these women were going through and the creative process gave participants permission to experience, articulate and animate their potential differently. The fluidity between visual and embodied practice as part of the clinical work supported the integration of differentiated and disparate aspects of individual and group processes, which themselves became a catalyst for change and transformation.

References

Bailly, L. (2009). *Lacan*. Oxford: Oneworld Publication.

Behm, M. (2022). Transformation across the art forms: Metamorphosis and motif. In Vaculik, C. & Nash, G. (eds.) *Integrative arts psychotherapy*. London: Routledge, Chapter 2. pp. 26–37.

Burrell, C. & Cohen, M. (2018). Moving colour: Combining Dance Movement Psychotherapy and art psychotherapy in a NHS community women's group. In Colbert, T. & Bent, C. (eds.) *Working across modalities in the arts therapies*. Oxon/New York: Routledge, pp. 15–29.

Claxton, G. (2015). *Intelligence in the flesh. Why your mind needs your body much more than it thinks*. New Haven/London: Yale University Press.

Colbert, T. & Bent, C. (2018). *Working across modalities in the arts therapies*. Oxon/New York: Routledge.

Grant, A. (2021). *There's a name for the blah you're feeling: It's called languishing*. The New York Times, April [available online at https://www.nytimes.com/2021/04/19/well/mind/covid-mental-health-languishing.html].

McNiff, S. (1998). *Trust the process, an artist's guide to letting go*. Boston & London: Shambhala.

Perry, G. (2021). Grayson's Art Club. Channel 4.

Rova, M., Burrell, C. & Cohen, M. (2020). Existing in-between two worlds: Supporting asylum seeking women living in temporary accommodation through a creative movement and art intervention. *Body, Movement and Dance in Psychotherapy: An International Journal for Theory, Research and Practice*, 15 (3), pp. 204–218.

Stern, D (2010). *Forms of vitality: Exploring dynamic experience in psychology, the arts, psychotherapy, and development*. Oxford: Oxford University Press.

Tempest, K. (2020). *On connection*. London: Faber.

Trevarthen, C. (1983). Emotions in infancy: Regulators of contacts and relationships with persons. In K. Scherer & Ekman, P. (eds.) *Approaches to emotion*, Hillsdale, NJ: Lawrence Erlbaum Associates, Inc. pp. 129–155.

Turner, V. (2017). *The ritual process: Structure and anti-structure*. New York & London: Routledge.

van Gennep, A. (1960). *The rites of passage*. London: Routledge & Kegan Paul.

Winnicott, D. (1971). *Playing and reality*. London & New York: Routledge.

15 Indominus Rex; developing mentalisation with offenders through externalisation and creativity in a Dance Movement Psychotherapy group

Dawn Batcup

Dance Movement Psychotherapists draw on many theories to support the furtherance of our own developing body of evidence and knowledge. Systemic and group theory is particularly relevant, as Dance Movement Psychotherapy (DMP) is often provided in groups. The development of reflective capacity or *mentalisation* (Bateman & Fonagy 2016) is also pivotal, given it refers to people's ability to understand what is going on in our own mind[1] and to see how this is inextricably linked to bodily feelings, emotions, senses, context, relationships and attachment story.

Personal stories may be told in both movement and words in DMP, often using metaphors, which are examples of externalisations that can add to the creative process and meaning making. This chapter will focus on externalisation in these ways, alongside developing mentalisation with a group of offenders detained in a Medium Secure Unit (MSU) under the Criminal Justice System and Mental Health System. Individualised blame and internalised pathology can be typically how offender populations are socially organised and systemically understood, which can lead them to internalise further unlovable and blameful versions of themselves. This chapter seeks to show how DMP can contribute to situating delinquency in a relational context, whilst considering violent behaviour as a communication and mentalisation collapse, which disturbingly externalises the hurt when people have felt wronged. It will argue further that communicating, putting out and externalising those unhelpful, internalised processes can also be meaningful and liberating, enabling the re-authoring of personal narratives and recovery of mentalising when contained within the psychotherapy relationship.

Externalisation entails focusing on the problem as the problem and not the person (White & Epston 1990). It comes from narrative approaches in systemic therapy, which capitalise on being curious about other people's stories (Burnham 2000). Ideologically, this can often seem at odds within organisational systems designed for discipline and correction. In this chapter, I will present a clinical vignette, which focuses on considering an MSU client for a DMP group and viewing his participation in it as he shares and makes helpful externalisations as part of the collective.

DOI: 10.4324/9781003222484-15

Clinical context

Receiving help and joining a group

To protect confidentiality, the client joining the group is called Blake, a 25-year-old white, English man and only child from working class parents. Blake was an MSU inpatient, where he had been detained for four years, regularly assaulting staff, a presenting problem that hinted at his primary problems. His DMP referral came from his Multi-Disciplinary Team, exasperated but hopeful that DMP's combination of non-verbal/verbal approach could help Blake overcome his violent tendencies and deepen understanding about its meaning (Batcup 2012).

I dreaded meeting Blake. His difficult demeanour and violent outbursts were well known throughout the Service. Unusually, I argued that he may not be a suitable DMP candidate and delayed meeting him. But, when we met, I warmed to Blake immediately, perceiving his physical awkwardness as not wanting to develop into his adult self. I was not expecting him to remind me of myself. My own attachment narrative was reignited, triggering my fondness for this unpopular patient, considered one of the most dangerous in the MSU. As a woman of a similar age to his mum, this may have also enabled me to see him as a son, which possibly mirrored how he may have seen me as a mother (Ramasubramanian & Batcup 2021), with the same skin colour and working class origins. These aspects drew attention to what was visibly similar between us, whilst our gender differences may have amplified the possibility for parent-child transferences.

As a mother, I was struggling with separating from my teenager going to University when I met Blake. His stubborn and opinionated demeanour and relentless arguments with the Team reminded me of relentless arguments with my daughter in the months before she left. I understood that the arguments communicated pain and anguish linked to the difficulty of leaving, separating and signposted a pivotal moment in family life cycles (Carter & McGoldrick 1989), which are extremely stressful, especially tormenting and almost indecipherable when attachment and separation was insensitively handled. Despite or perhaps because of the rapport that developed between Blake and me, the actual content of the conversation in our first meeting was mainly introductory, administrative and factual.

In the next meeting, after much empathetic listening to Blake complaining about living in an MSU, I introduced the idea of using movement. I invited him to stand with me, offering basic grounding movements (Sandel et al. 1993). Blake followed and his responses became belligerent as he cynically mimicked a sexualised dance form. I felt sad and hopeless, trusting that this may be relevant; I tapped the beat of his movements with my foot, attempting an open stance to attune to his feelings (Stern 1985).

'No!' Blake asserted. Assuming he meant me to stop moving, I paused.

'I have to get this to work for me' he offered. I asked what that might look like. He did not know. I suggested we take inspiration from the movement props in the room, purposely decreasing the intensity between us by utilising an object through which we might connect through more safely (Novy et al. 2005). Blake was interested in the array of objects on the shelf but particularly drawn to the fabrics. He wrapped himself in a couple of these and took another to share with me. The fabrics he wore seemed to provide him with an extra protective layer, akin perhaps to the skin as a container (Bick 1968) whilst the larger fabric he shared with me represented the space between us and our relationship. A rhythm developed and a delicate dance emerged involving us both, with subtle twists that sustained the connection whilst freeing and binding the tension flow (Laban 1960) which I tried to reflect empathetically.

'What now?' Blake asked.

Keen not to rush him and valuing the nascent creative process, I followed his verbalisation and suggested we talk about what emerged in the movement. Blake talked about feeling silly but having a strange impulse to cry. He talked about his bewilderment regarding how his life had turned out the way it had, mentioning with embarrassment what he called 'the incident', referencing the offence that had brought him into detention. Blake was keen to proceed with DMP, his curiosity now triggered about his own internal processes and relationship issues. I offered him a place in a newly established mixed sex DMP group comprising others from the MSU, which I conducted on a weekly basis with a male co-worker.

I discovered from Blake's notes that his parents had died in their late fifties, in a road traffic accident shortly before he committed the offence that brought him into Forensic Services. Since offending, he was disowned by the extended family. He rarely mentioned them and has no next of kin recorded in the National Health Service records system. Blake's offence involved snatching a crying baby from its seemingly disinterested mother in order to soothe it. I was interested in the multiple meanings of what the offence might communicate (Cecchin 1987), but did not ask him about it in initial meetings, alluding instead to being interested too in how his life had unfolded in the way it had. Being deeply moved by Blake's desperate and uncontrollable urge to soothe a distressed baby and punish a carer, I considered his offence as a mirror to the impact and consequences of the often unbearable distress within insecure attachment (Ainsworth & Bowlby 1965).

Attachment and systems

Psychotherapy for offenders on an individual basis was deemed ineffective when it was noticed how, when people returned to their families, delinquent behaviours re-emerged, suggesting the problems may be in the family and not in the individual (Minuchin et al. 1967). But, what if there is no family available to work with, as in Blake's case? This aloneness is not unusual for Forensic clients, typically diagnosed with anti-social and/or borderline personality disorders. Adshead (1998) writes about psychiatric staff as attachment figures and from this, it may be possible to consider behavioural patterns in the ward as communications to extend curiosity about what Blake may have internalised about himself, his family, care, attachment and relationships.

Attachment refers to our earliest bonds and experiences of receiving care, help and protection. Within secure attachments, babies turn to their attachment figures when distressed, communicate this and receive soothing (Bowlby 1988 & 1999). Those who have experienced secure attachments internalise this process and learn that their feelings are valid, bearable and understandable. They go on to be confident in their understanding of themselves, their emotions and in making healthy relationships for and with themselves. Blake, like others in the DMP group, had not had secure attachment experiences growing up. Instead, he experienced severe neglect, adversity and violence at the hands of his parents and was known to social services as a safeguarding concern. As a troubled teenager, Blake's foster placements often broke down and he regularly changed homes and schools, which is not an unusual pattern for Forensic clients.

Breaking down and breaking through

Blake made a serious commitment to the weekly DMP group and in the first three months, rarely missed a session. Dalal (1998) referring to Foulkes writes about group affiliation as quintessential to the process of rehabilitation, which is more pressing where there has been insecure attachment, isolation, problems with authority and delinquency which intensifies desires for gang affiliation (Nitsun, 1996).

But Blake's aggression in the Unit escalated again. Troubled by therapy breaks, his former defences and strategies about needing no one seemed to be breaking down. His aggression was such he was stopped from attending sessions. It seemed important for me to 'fight' for his return to the group behind the scenes, debating assertively with his Team to bring him to sessions, particularly when the acting out was troublesome and that this was when he needed sessions most. A compromise was found: Blake was escorted to sessions by Unit staff but had to wear plastic handcuffs whilst a staff member sat outside the therapy room. Normally, all staff wear alarms and there are alarms on the session room wall.

Group members were relieved when Blake attended again. They updated him on what he had missed and were keen to hear how he had coped with the added restrictions. The group never questioned his decisions to lash out, instead they were fervently aligned in their sense of injustice; 'Just walk away, mate' offered another, Stanley, a black man in his fifties who had attempted suicide in prison during his long sentence for illicit drug dealing and gang related violence.

Envisioning Blake walking away and putting space not violence between himself and another made me keen to open an imaginable space for creative exploration between the group's perceptions of injustice and aggressive reactions. I tried an externalising intervention (Burnham 2000; White & Epston, 1990) to find new ways to understand the violence. I empathetically asked Blake what it might look like if he were to take this thing, this feeling or sense, outside of himself, whilst gesturing with my hands as if trying to hold or grapple with something tangible. Blake looked at me, frowned and appeared puzzled. I looked at him, empathetically reflecting his puzzlement whilst feeling incompetent, assuming he would not respond further. There was a silent but pregnant pause that I resisted filling.

> Then, to my astonishment, Blake said "Indominus Rex".
> "What's that?" I responded, genuinely not understanding.
> "Indominus Rex", he repeated, smiling playfully "it's a dinosaur!"
> I listened as Blake enlightened the group with a detailed account of this dinosaur's nature and appearance, which also gave way to dialogue, where we could be curious and ask more questions. In his responses, Blake seemed freer and said, "That's easy".

An animated discussion flowed between the group members led by Blake: The dinosaur being a helpful externalisation for impulsive, over-reactive, aggressive and non-mentalising behaviours, with which Blake's peers resonated. Here, it would seem that the externalisation began to enable the group to overcome the defence against thinking about itself (Bion 1961) and instead, the members managed to inquire into their groupness alongside an inquiry into the workings of the mind. Hopper (2002) discussed how the group can be used as an object for collective transference for domains held in common. Perhaps the group members were exploring aspects of deeply held prejudices and projections about criminality, in this instance, symbolised by a cold-blooded animal, the dinosaur. I thought that they could have also been exploring how their interpersonal modus operandi and their failed attempts at closeness were outdated and like dinosaurs, extinct. I put my thoughts aside but asked the group questions previously considered too provoking, concerning when dinosaurs first arrived in people's lives and what the MSU Teams are doing when it is causing most or least trouble. Previously, without the dinosaur externalisation, details of individual miscommunication events and subtle mis-attunements made group members lose the thread. I asked about the impact the dinosaur's presence had on the Team and the Team's impact on the dinosaur's presence at varying times and most importantly, we established that there were times when the dinosaur was not there.

Blake referred to his parent's attempt to suffocate him when he was a child and how the dinosaur causes mayhem when he recalls this with the Team. He voiced that 'they' do not take this or the damage it caused seriously, which amplified the group's belief that 'they' do not care. Asking sensitively about who were 'they' and what that reminded people about, Penny replied. She was a woman in her late twenties who had been trafficked from Eastern Europe and had attempted to strangle the baby conceived non-consentingly following sex for payment. She made a link to early experiences of her own depressed mother who did not care and an essentially absent father not focused on her at her most vulnerable time. Others in the group did not know her offence but understood that she was fighting to see her baby and had previously obeyed instructions from voices she heard. They fretfully questioned if they should be holding onto this, or letting it go.

Emotions were high in the room. The participants appeared restless as they looked at each other and glimpsed back at their early neglect, re-experiencing the unkind words spoken and the hurt feelings felt from long ago. I carefully made a transition into movement to reflect people's bodily cues, emotions and themes regarding their verbal theme of holding onto or letting go, which I turned into a non-verbal opening and closing of hands. This movement intervention brought people into closer proximity as they became fascinated by how the same thing could be done so differently. This had resonance with Yalom's (2005) idea about interpersonal learning in the group concerning similarity and difference. Being together with others and similar whilst also being different was clearly seen in the hand movements. Building from dinosaurs, I spoke about the protective function of instincts for survival, offering protection against threat, be that real or imagined. In expanding the curiosity, I suggested that we used movement props to build safe spaces for ourselves in the room. People hurried to the movement props on the shelf, gathered materials for their constructions and busied themselves with their creations. Carefully laid yoga blocks, fabrics and cushions now demarcated and subdivided the floor area around each individual. After moving in and around their own symbolic homes, they were curious to visit each other's, respectful to not enter unless asked.

In reflecting back verbally on the movement from within their crafted spaces, Blake started, saying he noticed Indominus Rex was currently absent. When asked what it was in the movement that may have enabled this, Blake made a link to the act of exploration, curiosity and building safe spaces, admitting that when the MSU Team were curious, the Unit could sometimes be a safe place too. He spoke highly of his relationship with the Team in these moments. This was the first time he had talked about having a good relationship with the Team. Others in the group found examples of MSU Team members being therapeutic, and empathy for staff took shape in a discussion of how hard it must be to be a nurse. Blake was excited as he and the group excavated an important *difference*, an exception to what he and the group considered the norm about people who don't care, which was significant in the unfolding therapeutic collective narrative.

Exploring this as a 'unique outcome' (White & Epston 1990) took up the remainder of the session. The idea was entertained that care might not always be punishing and that the past did not always have to wreak havoc in the future. Enthused, Blake humorously added how Indominus Rex's upper limbs were too short to reach out and make physical contact with another. He gestured to his own wrists, disclosing that they were restricted by the plastic handcuffs which he had expertly tucked under his sleeves. It was a relief that the humour subsided and we stayed silent in the emotionally painful moment together.

Endings

In ending the group, Blake's peer offered that we, us people, unlike dinosaurs, could communicate and rely on others, such as therapists and the MSU Team, when our own reflective capacity was adversely affected. I agreed, mentioning that the group seemed to be exploring interdependence, nurturing and contemplating that whilst it might not be fully possible to leave the past behind us, we did not have to let it shape the future. I thought that this was a breakthrough.

It was noteworthy that Blake was handcuff free when escorted to sessions from then on. He became a respected group member, active in contributing to creative ideas which led to understanding how we may inadvertently contribute to the maintenance of problems and or preventing change. Blake was pivotal in using movement to support meaning making which led to being seen, listened to, challenged and disagreed with. Gradually, as blame and shame reduced, the primary task became to understand how problems became embedded, internalised and acted out. The need for interventions that made direct externalisations of *the problem* became less pressing and communication abilities grew whilst violence receded. The gap left by family no longer needed to be filled with objects and could now be open to allow space for other people and ideas. The group began to question socio economic stressors and how we are organised alongside the impact of family dynamics, intergenerational trauma, attachment trauma, ethnicity, gender and sexuality. In the group, there was also acknowledgement that whilst we may not always get it right with understanding and attuning to each other but that we were there, to try and to remain curious, which was probably a new experience for them.

Blake's story is unique but not totally unlike other people who offend. It was probably not coincidental that his detainment came soon after his parent's death, leading him to a Forensic Institution rather than University, his offence being a behavioural response to disorganised insecure attachment patterns reactivated by a harsh and unpredicted attachment separation (Vetere & Dallos 2008). Like others in his situation, the traumatic impact of insecure attachment seems to have been replayed in his offence and echoed in current relationships. According to Minuchin (1984), structures tend to self-perpetuate when there is negative feedback from the system or organisation. Blake's re-enactments towards carers inadvertently showed how 'care' had hurt him. In response, MSU staff felt hopeless, unable to help and turned to medication and seclusion, which further amplified Blake's feelings of neglect and anger towards authority, a process typical with offenders (Ruszczynski 2010). However, DMP may be beginning to provide Blake with a secure base (Bowlby 1988) within which to explore and build a coherent narrative, alongside experiencing me, the group and Unit staff as a maternal-parental attachment that will not hurt him.

Conclusion

In focusing on the variety of theories DMP can draw upon to inform practice, systemic and group theory provided the context for the externalisation and mentalising interventions and this enabled the group to overcome the defence against thinking about itself and each other in context. The findings in this case study being that externalisation can be most effective as part of an embodied creative process.

Relationship issues need reliable relationships for recovery and understanding that to better know one's own mind, it can be the receptive and attuned mind of another (Stern 1985) or *marked mirroring* (Bateman & Fonagy 2016) that can help. The group situation was also crucial in the context of the vignette, as we see Blake being confronted with various aspects of himself reflected from different perspectives and angles, like a 'hall of mirrors' (Foulkes & Anthony, 1957: 150).

From the start, movement processes revealed Blake's significant distress through symbolism and rhythm, which also supported our nascent therapeutic relationship and perhaps also helped him access the group. Yalom (2005) talked about the group as a good place for the repetition and repair of family dynamic issues. In the absence of family and secure attachments, groups may also be the best places to find kindness, compassion and protection from being drawn into gang membership.

The practice and knowledge of DMP can make a valuable contribution within a medico-legal MSU context. Whilst being literally locked in, there may be an ideological tension in considering the problem as the problem and not the person, but there is also the opportunity and time for people to embark authentically upon discovering an internal freedom from defence mechanisms, distress and trauma to break through the sociocultural and less conscious restraints that construct and organise us all.

Note

1 By "mind" the author follows Siegal (2012), meaning the embodied, embedded, emergent and relational process that both tracks and transforms.

References

Adshead, G. (1998). Psychiatric staff as attachment figures. *British Journal of Psychiatry*, 17 (2), pp. 64–69.

Ainsworth, M. & Bowlby, J. (1965). *Child care and the growth of love*. London: Penguin.

Batcup, D. (2012). A discussion of the DMP literature relative to prisons and medium secure units Body. *Movement and Dance in Psychotherapy: An International Journal for Theory, Research & Practice*, 8 (1), pp. 5–16.

Bateman, A. & Fonagy, P. (2016). *Mentalization based therapy for personality disorders.* London: OU Press.

Bick, E. (1968). The experience of the skin in early object relations. *International Journal of Psychoanalysis,* 49, pp. 484–486.

Bion, W. (1961). *Experiences in groups.* London: Routledge.

Bowlby, J. (1988). *A secure base: parent-child attachment & healthy human development. Tavistock Professional Books.* London: Routledge.

Bowlby, J. (1999). (2nd edition). *Attachment. Attachment and Loss* (vol. 1). New York: Basic Books.

Burnham, B. (2000). Internalised other interviewing: evaluation and enhancing empathy. *Clinical Psychology Forum,* 140, pp. 16–20.

Carter, B. & McGoldrick, M. (eds.) (1989). *The changing family life cycle: a framework for family therapy.* Boston & London: Allyn & Bacon.

Cecchin, G. (1987). Hypothesising, circularity and neutrality revisited: an invitation to curiosity. *Family Processes,* 26 (4), pp. 405–413.

Dalal, F. (1998). *Towards a post Foulksian analysis; taking the group seriously.* London: Blackwell.

Foulkes, S.H. & Anthony, E.J. (1957). *Group psychotherapy; the psycho-analytic approach.* London: Penguin.

Hopper, E. (2002). *The social unconscious.* London: Jessica Kingsley.

Laban, R. (1960). *The mastery of movement.* 2nd edition. Macdonald & Evans: London: Northcote House.

Minuchin, S. (1984). *Family kaleidoscope.* Cambridge/London: Harvard.

Minuchin, S., Montalvo, R., Guerney, B., Rosman, B. & Schumer, F. (1967). *Families of the slums.* New York: Basic Books.

Nitsun, M. (1996). *The anti group; destructive forces in the group and their creative potential.* London, New York: Routledge.

Novy, C., Ward, S., Thomas, A., Bulmer, L. & Gauthier, M. (2005). Introducing movement and prop as additional metaphors in narrative therapy. *Journal of Systemic Therapies,* 24 (2), pp. 60–74.

Ramasubramanian, P. & Batcup, D. (2021). Exploring maternal and erotic transference in DMP with a sex offender. In Hastilow, S. & Leibmann, M. (eds.) *Arts Therapies and Sexual Offending.* London: Jessica Kingsley, pp. 79–96.

Ruszczynski, S. (2010). Becoming neglected: a perverse relationship to care. *British Journal of Psychotherapy,* 26 (1), pp. 22–32.

Sandel, S. et al. (1993). *Foundations of dance/movement therapy: the life and work of Marian Chace.* Columbia, MD: The Marian Chace Memorial Fund of the American Dance Therapy Association.

Siegal, D. (2012). *Pocket guide to interpersonal neurobiology: an integrated hand book of the mind.* New York/London: Norton.

Stern, D. (1985). *The interpersonal world of the infant. A view from psychoanalysis and developmental psychology.* New York: Basic Books.

Vetere, A. & Dallos, R. (2018). Systemic theory and attachment narratives: attachment narrative therapy. *Journal of Family Therapy,* 30 (4), pp. 371–385.

White, M. & Epston, D. (1990). *Narrative means to therapeutic ends.* Dulwich Centre Newsletter.

Yalom, I. (2005). *The theory and practice of group psychotherapy,* 5th edition. New York: Perseus Book.

16 Dancing with Stephen

Reconnecting with the body in a search for closure

Goretti Barjacoba-Souto

As a dance movement psychotherapist working with children with profound and complex needs in school settings, I know facing the loss of a client is not an uncommon event and one I have encountered more than once. Despite years of experience, personal therapy and supervision, I still find tears rolling down my face as I write these words. As a mother I acknowledge this is a particularly sensitive subject that deeply touches my own personal experience, as I closely faced the possible death of a child of my own a few years ago and this has been an area for ongoing work and development in my self-healing journey.

In this chapter, it is not my intention to engage in an in-depth discussion about loss and bereavement. I seek to share my experiential process to find meaning and closure after the death of a child with whom I worked. Even though our sessions had come to an end months before his death, it still had a profound effect on me, particularly due to the timing and circumstances around it.

After the summer of 2020, I went back to work in a Special Educational Needs and Disabilities (SEND) school where I have been employed for a number of years. That was when I heard that Stephen, a child I had worked with before, had passed away a few months earlier. I had not been to the school in six months due to the Covid-19 pandemic and that was not the kind of news I was expecting when I arrived with the excitement of seeing everyone again after the long break. Under different circumstances, the school would have come together to celebrate his life and honour his memory, but the restrictions in place due to Coronavirus meant that would not be possible. While I understood why these restrictions were in place, I still struggled with feelings of sadness, frustration and anger.

My own movement practice and supervision allowed me to process the experience and deal with my emotions to a certain extent. However, they did not seem enough. Near the first anniversary of Stephen's death, I allowed my grieving body to dance moving my memories of our work. I thought of his parents' pain and just like a mother refusing to let go of a beloved child, I did not want his name to be forgotten and memories of his life to disappear, so I decided to write about my work and relationship with Stephen.

DOI: 10.4324/9781003222484-16

Being a very personal and intimate experience, I chose to address my words to Stephen directly, knowing that I wanted to share them with his parents too. Then, whilst I was immersed in that process, I realised that sharing my writing with others who knew him in the school that he attended would be a great opportunity to remember and celebrate him, but also a chance to share a more profound perspective of my work within that setting. Stephen's parents not only gave me permission to do so, but they also asked me to use his real name and to take things even further, to publish the story, so now you can read about Stephen here. For that reason, his name has not been anonymised in this chapter.

First, I would like to clarify and acknowledge that the use of touch is an essential element in my work with most children with profound and multiple learning disabilities, both to provide support and as a therapeutic intervention. I believe that touch is a natural element in most relationships, but how can I mindfully and ethically integrate it in my work?

Although an in-depth discussion on this subject is beyond the scope of this chapter, it is important to bear in mind that this is a controversial aspect in psychotherapy and ethical considerations must be taken into account. Some therapists argue that touch can elicit different responses, including sexual, power and aggressive connotations, and it is not appropriate for all clients (Popa & Best 2010; Westland 2011; Zur 2008).

Many authors have argued that the use of touch is extremely beneficial for some clients (Butté & Unkovich 2009; Gale & Hegarty 2000; Hartley 2004; Popa & Best 2010; Kestenberg, Loman & Sossin 1999). In fact, touch appears to be linked to early life experiences, brain development, sense of self, secure attachment, communication, self-regulation and even the formation of the therapeutic alliance (Bainbridge Cohen 2018; Dymoke 2019; Popa & Best 2010; Westland 2011). Westland (2011) also listed other benefits related to the release of hormones stimulated through touch, like lifting mood, reducing anxiety, pain relief, as well as the reduction in muscle tension, to name just a few.

In my work setting, the official guidelines allow *proper physical contact* to support students. The need for cuddles or close contact is also acknowledged and recommended in those situations when the child requires it, as long as it is *carried out sensitively* within public view.

I have observed that in our Western society adults tend to use touch with children more freely than with other adults, often without much consideration for the child's opinions. Of course, cultural differences come into play here, but coming from a Mediterranean culture, I clearly remember that as a child I was expected to greet distant relatives with a kiss or a hug, even when that did not feel right to me. Today, I still hold on to those memories and when I interact with children I want to show them the same respect I would show another adult, particularly when it comes to physical boundaries.

With all this in mind, given Stephen's physical limitations, in our sessions I provided physical support to mobilise his limbs or help him change position.

I also used props to massage different body parts to relax them, or bring his awareness to them, in preparation for a free creative self-expression. However, as a way of showing respect and to anticipate the next step, I would verbalise what I was about to do and sought signs that could indicate any discomfort or disagreement with my actions, as Stephen was not able to express consent verbally. I regularly reminded him to let me know if something did not feel right and suggested options, like making a sound or pulling away. This communication felt extremely important to me, as I knew that throughout the day his body would often be moved by those supporting him (or attending to his needs). Even when care is given with the best intentions, there is still a risk of objectifying someone's body when attending to their physical needs. Hence, the importance of treating Stephen with the same respect I would demonstrate to an independent able-bodied adult.

Stephen

I find myself alone in my living room, a light and airy space. Standing facing a large window, I stare at the sky. I see some clouds, the sun and big trees. The sunrays entering the room appear to be flooding the space whilst a turmoil of emotions start flooding my body. I take a deep breath, shut my eyes and stand tall, noticing my bare feet grounded on the wooden floor. Unable to move, I take a few more breaths and gradually these breaths guide my body out of that position. Light delicate movements start in my fingers and gently travel to the rest of my body. I think about you, Stephen, and find myself looking for a way to say goodbye. While I dance, I meet feelings of sadness, frustration and disempowerment. A few minutes pass. I find my way to the floor, where I lie enjoying the support the ground is offering and I achieve a sense of release while tears flow down my face. Some things can feel so unfair and I wish I could make them better. After a few deep breaths, I remember the serenity prayer: *God, grant me the serenity to accept the things I cannot change; Courage to change the things I can; And wisdom to know the difference.*

Our journey began over three years ago when you were four and started attending the DMP sessions I facilitated for some children in your class. A year later, we began to meet for individual sessions. One of the first things I noticed about you was your beautiful round face and big dark eyes. A handsome boy with a four-limb motor disorder that caused involuntary constant twitching and jerking, as well as a limited range of movement. Your facial expression seemed always unchanged, which like a foreign tongue, I could not read. For a while it was a challenge, until I learnt to notice the most subtle shifts in the corners of your mouth and the quiet language of your eyes.

Our sessions began with a short hello song and a check-in, using the body to share our emotional state. Next, the focus was to bring awareness to the different parts with a whole body warm up. This felt particularly important, because as MacDonald (1992) explains, 'many people with learning difficulties have great problems with relating to their own bodies and recognising body parts' (206). While you were lying on a mat, I wondered about your perception of your own physical boundaries and I used physical contact to develop your kinaesthetic awareness[1] (Levy 1992; Whitehouse 1999). With balls and bean bags I massaged and tried to encourage your muscles to relax. Gradually, I encouraged a shift of attention to the joints, easing them, to gently expand their range of movement. I remember my excitement observing the impact of the warm up. I used to start gently but actively moving your body, stretching your limbs in different directions, testing the movement range that was available to your joints, making circles, opening and closing, exploring and expanding your kinesphere. I could clearly feel how it was becoming easier and easier, as your body started to loosen and you needed less support from me, until we would slowly begin to move together sharing the leading role. Then, depending on your energy levels, some days I would simply provide gentle support while you were able to lead me into your dance almost completely, while I followed your non-verbal cues. These achievements were positive steps towards developing confidence and self-esteem (Levy 1992).

As we continued our creative exploration, we would play with a variety of props, which you were able to choose by looking at your preferred one, when I held a couple of them up close to your eyes. Encouraging you to make choices was important, as a way of empowering you and contributing to your sense of self-worth, particularly considering that throughout your life many of your decisions were made by others (Chesner, 1995). Pompons were one of your favourites, but we also enjoyed a shared experience with scarves, stretchy cloths, balls and musical instruments. We used to explore different ways of expressing ourselves, engaging, creating and being playful.

As you did not communicate verbally, and I was not able to rely on your facial expressions, I searched for alternatives, focusing on embodied communication during our exchanges. In order for me to gauge your emotional and physical state, my own body served me as a vessel to feel and understand what was happening in yours. As Clark & Smith (2017) state 'through recognising the subtle differences that arise at a physical level when working with someone who has little or no verbal communication, we hone into a deeper sense of connection with our own body and that of our client and step into the physicality of the communication with them' (Clark & Smith 2017: 114). While I focused on my embodied intuition, our bodies and movement were our shared language. I noticed my own somatic responses carefully, as well as any subtle changes in yours to guide us through our sessions. The key for me was to stay present in the here and now, to attune and mirror as a way of reflecting back and responding to you using our physical connection (Clark & Smith 2017).

Similarly to Butté's (2017) approach, I used to share my own feelings with you when I felt that they could be a reflection of your own.

> In my work with clients whose communication is predominantly non-verbal, I share my own feelings; feelings that I believe are theirs which

I am intuitively, somatically or emotionally resonating with; and the feelings that would be natural for many of us in a given situation – those that are part of our collective human experience. I do this in order to let my clients know that we indeed all have feelings and that no feelings are taboo (Butté, 2017:138).

With time I discovered that when I was looking for confirmation of a concept or an idea, your eyes could also offer an answer to queries that I verbalised. By asking you to make eye contact to acknowledge, or move your eyes away to refuse or deny something, you offered answers to simple questions. That was particularly helpful when I wanted to know if you were uncomfortable or in pain. Other times, we used the same pattern with picture cards with various choices, so you could select one out of two. That also became useful at the beginning and the end of the sessions, so you could choose a card that reflected how you felt to check-in and out. The emphasis on those abilities was another way of giving you a voice, feeding your sense of empowerment.

At times, I noticed my insecurities and felt unsure of your interpretation of my words, but then I also witnessed your effort to apply my suggestions to reach some of our movement goals more easily and efficiently. As you spent most hours of your day in a wheelchair, one of my objectives was to give your body freedom to move without the constrictions of that chair, to stretch, to explore the boundaries of your skin, expand your kinesphere and bring awareness to all your body parts, as well as discovering new ways of moving. On the other hand, I did not want you to be a passive recipient of my interventions. I also wanted to give you a *voice*, the power to make decisions, choices, to express yourself and be heard. As a result, I aimed to create a safe space for any difficult or painful feelings, but also a place for you to have enjoyable and positive embodied experiences. As Frizell (2017) noted: 'The ability to attune on an embodied level and to mirror the affective essence of the client's story opens opportunities for the therapist to experience and understand the transference and for the client and to feel heard, seen and understood' (16).

Despite the physical limitations, I observed your movement range increase slightly, particularly your arm movements that were slowly expanding, and your willingness to try new things. Facilitating enjoyable movement experiences offers the opportunity to understand that the 'negative experiences are only one aspect' (Papadopoulos, 2015: 4) of someone's life and it is also possible to connect with 'enjoyable aspects of themselves' (ibid). Even though Papadopoulos (2015) writes specifically about people who experience different psychological difficulties, I believe her views are relevant here, as simple exercises can result in changes in someone's mood and enable a transformational experience. These positive experiences of change through the body can help to counteract negative experiences and translate into a sense of purpose and agency that goes beyond the therapeutic (Papadopolous 2015; Sheets-Johnstone 2010).

Winter months took a toll on your body. The impact on your health was obvious and I could see your effort to breathe. Your cough was a real struggle, and the worry in your eyes became clear. Changing your position on the mat offered a temporary relief. However, I was still left with my own feelings of frustration and disempowerment, as I wanted to make you better. At times, the exhaustion took over your body and you fell asleep during our sessions. Then I would become your witness while allowing your body to rest, welcoming whatever it needed. I would adjust my expectations to meet you in the moment. After those meetings, I often heard well-meaning comments saying: 'What a shame he missed part of his session!' To which I explained that we should accept and respect that was what your body needed. Working in a goal oriented setting, it may be difficult for a therapist to accept the need and importance of just simply sitting and being present with a client, witnessing what is happening in the moment, rather than doing something (Butté 2017). I felt you trusted me to share your journey and those moments of stillness were as valuable to me as those when I cheered your achievements and our discoveries with pride.

I had the honour of being part of your journey for two years. I am proud of the moments we shared and grateful for everything you taught me from our work together. I know at times you were happy, while others less so. We had moments when you must have been uncomfortable, perhaps frustrated, angry or sad. Once more, I reflect back on the serenity prayer. Even though I accept that I could not cure your body, I also believe I was able to make some moments better and offer some healing during our time together. Now I can also say that navigating through this process, dancing with your memories and writing about our journey, I found courage and wisdom to deeply embody and understand both the things I could not change and those that I could. Stephen, I would like to think that you felt you were heard, that you felt met, supported and understood. I also wonder if I was able to touch your soul, because you definitely touched my own.

Closing dance

After putting my experience with Stephen in writing, sharing it with those close to him and writing this chapter, I decided once again to go back to my starting point and to reconnect with my body. Back in the same room where my grieving body started this dance, I stand still and allow the experience to lead me in movement one more time. When I look outside, I see the first signs of autumn. Like the leaves of some trees that are beginning to fall saying goodbye to the branches that held them since the spring, I start to say goodbye to this piece of writing that was born from the seed of an embodied exploration. In seeking closure, dancing seems the best way to end this journey. I close my eyes and visualise Stephen's face. Slowly I feel like my body is melting all the way down and I find myself crouching into a small ball with my hands hiding my face. I stay there for a moment before lying on the cold floor. I enjoy the support that the ground offers, which slowly starts to warm up from the contact with my body. Taking a deep breath, I notice a sensation of fullness and satisfaction in my stomach. I stay there for a while and then, allow my breath to move me. Very slowly my head starts to turn from side to side and gradually the movement travels down my spine to the rest of the body. I continue the dance for a few minutes, not completely aware of time. I enjoy opening and closing movements, rolling from one side of my body and then, to the other. Soon, I realise that I am mirroring a dance that Stephen and I used to do together. I am drawing big arm circles, with one arm at a time, first opening to the side and then slowly moving upwards, stretching up around beyond my head and then coming down the opposite side where my arm meets my torso, with the rest of my body following until I roll completely to one side. Then I reverse the movement rolling to the other side, shifting back and forth, from left to right and right to left. I enjoy feeling my body fully stretching in the middle facing up, before completing the circle to the side where I curl up. Eventually I pause. I stay lying down on the floor facing up, with my legs hip-width apart. My arms are stretched over my head making a V-shape. Slowly they begin to relax and bend at the elbows, before finding my chest. I take a deep breath and a smile appears on my face. I finally feel ready to let go. A sense of profound gratitude fills my body and I feel at peace.

Conclusion

Sue Curtis (2017) explains the importance of having a good plan in place in school settings to provide bereavement support when facing the death of a student. However, the circumstances around the loss of Stephen meant that we did not have the chance to work through this bereavement in the same way we would have in other circumstances (without the Covid-19 restrictions). I agree with Curtis (2017) that even though supervision plays a crucial role for therapists grappling with difficult feelings around loss and grief, just as I experienced after Stephen's death, focusing on the theory is not enough.

Loss is a bodily felt experience and grieving involves unconscious processes (Curtis 2017; Grey 2010). Rational thinking on its own was not enough to find resolution and closure without an embodied experience. When I listened to my body, allowing it to move, I tapped into my creativity to explore my responses towards Stephen's death. I was, therefore, able to access and make sense of thoughts and feelings that were previously hidden. Working from the inside out, using movement and creative writing to externalise the narrative of my embodied experience, I was able to bring the unconscious into my awareness and work through what otherwise would have remained trapped in my body as unresolved grief. Furthermore, the process guided me into making sense and integrating all aspects of my experience, allowing me to celebrate Stephen's life, find closure and move on.

As I previously mentioned, in this chapter it was not my objective to engage in an analysis of bereavement, loss and grief. Instead, my purpose was to share how my very personal exploration helped me transform pain and discomfort into learning, growth and fulfilment. Movement and writing were the vehicles that took my grieving body on a creative journey to find healing and gave a voice to a story that wanted to be heard. As in many other past experiences, once again, my moving creative body provided the unique and vital resources I needed to navigate the deep, unpredictable sea of loss and grief until I reached a safe ground.

In loving memory of Stephen Sopade

Note

1 Mary Whitehouse defined kinaesthetic awareness as the internal sense of someone's physical self, their ability to make a subjective connection with how it feels to move a certain way (Whitehouse 1999). It can also be described as an individual's ability to connect body and mind, tapping into his/her inner wisdom.

References

Bainbridge Cohen, B. (2018). *The basic neurocellular patterns, exploring developmental movement*. El Sobrante: Burchfield Rose.

Butté, C. (2017). How can I meet Syon where he is today? In Unkovich, G., Butté, C. & Butler, J. (eds.). *Dance Movement Psychotherapy with People with Learning Disabilities*. London: Routledge, pp. 136–147.

Butté, C. & Unkovich, G. (2009). Foundations of Dance Movement Psychotherapy practice in profound and multiple learning disabilities. *When Disabilities Disappear, e-Motion*, Vol. XIX, pp. 25–33.

Chesner, A. (1995). *Dramatherapy for people with learning disabilities. A world of difference*. London: Jessica Kingsley.

Clark, L. & Smith, V. (2017). I will dance with you, all that you have been, all that you are, and all that you can become: An exploration of the application of a person centred Dance Movement Psychotherapy approach with nonverbal clients in a group context. In Unkovich, G., Butté, C. & Butler, J. (eds.). *Dance Movement Psychotherapy with People with Learning Disabilities*. London: Routledge. pp. 109–120.

Curtis, S. (2017). On becoming a monkey. In Unkovich, G., Butté, C. & Butler, J. (eds.). *Dance Movement Psychotherapy with People with Learning Disabilities*. London: Routledge. pp. 81–93.

Dymoke, K. (2019). Touching the untouchables. Psychotherapy. Politics International, Wiley Online Library (accessed via https://onlinelibrary.wiley.com/doi/epdf/10.1002/ppi.1506 on 10/09/2021).

Frizell, C. (2017). Entering the world: Dance Movement Psychotherapy and the complexity of beginnings with learning disabled clients. In Unkovich, G., Butté, C. & Butler, J. (eds.). *Dance Movement Psychotherapy with People with Learning Disabilities*. London: Routledge, pp. 9–21.

Gale, E. & Hegarty, J.R. (2000). The use of touch in caring for people with learning disability. *British Journal of Learning Disabilities*, Vol. 46(2), pp. 97–108.

Grey, R. (2010). *Bereavement, loss and learning disabilities: A guide for professionals and carers*. London: Jessica Kingsley.

Hartley, L. (2004). *Somatic psychology: Body, mind, and meaning*. London: Whurr Publishing.

Kestenberg, A., Loman, S. & Sossin, K.M. (1999). *The meaning of movement: Developmental and clinical perspectives of the Kestenberg Movement Profile*. New York: Routledge.

Levy, F. (1992). *Dance movement therapy. A healing art*. Reston, VA: American Alliance for Health, Physical Education, Recreation and Dance.

MacDonald, J. (1992). Dance? Of course I can! dance movement therapy for people with learning difficulties. In Payne, H. (ed.). *Dance movement therapy: Theory and practice*. London: Routledge, pp. 202–217.

Sheets-Johnstone, M. (2010). Kinesthetic experience: Understanding movement inside and out. *In Body, Movement and Dance in Psychotherapy: An International Journal for Theory, Research and Practice*, Vol. 5(2), pp. 111–127.

Papadopoulos, N. (2015). The body as home. *E-motion ADMP UK*, Vol. XXV(3), pp. 4–7.

Popa, M.R. & Best, P.A. (2010). Making sense of touch in dance movement therapy: A trainee's perspective. In *Body, Movement and Dance In Psychotherapy: An International Journal for Theory, Research and Practice*, Vol. 5(1), pp. 31–44.

Westland, G. (2011). Physical touch in psychotherapy: Why are we not touching more? *In Body Movement and Dance in Psychotherapy: An International Journal for Theory, Research and Practice*, Vol. 6(11), pp. 17–29.

Whitehouse, M. (1999). Physical movement and personality. In Pallaro, P. (ed.). *Authentic movement: Essays by Mary Starks whitehouse, Janet Adler, and Joan Chodorow*. London: Jessica Kingsley, pp. 51–57.

Zur, O. (2008). Ethical and legal aspects of touch in psychotherapy. Zur Institute (accessed online via www.zurichinstitute.com/ethics-of-touch/).

17 The matriarch and the mollusc and all things in between

Caroline Frizell and Helen Poynor

This chapter has grown out of a peer collaboration which has evolved over some years both in the studio and in environments on Dartmoor and the Jurassic Coast in East Devon. It offers a window on our peer exchange as two mature women, both Dance Movement Psychotherapy practitioners, supervisors and educators. We meet three or four times a year for shared movement practice indoors and outdoors. The title of this chapter, 'the matriarch and the mollusc' is a feminist statement about our relationship navigated over the years, within the entangled intra-connectedness of all things, from the powerful matriarch to the soft bodied mollusc. Keen to maintain the primacy of movement in our process, this writing cobbles together fragments of our encounters, allowing themes of power, hierarchy, privilege and the materiality of moving bodies to seep in and out of the cracks of our reality. We invite you to accompany us through moments of moving, imagining, listening, musing and witnessing, within a psychic and emotional container of experience and skills strong enough to hold our own and the other's raw, unbridled expression.

Orienting

Polarised energies meet on a mat. One ready to go; needing to be witnessed and to be heard, a chaotic energy yearning to find form. An urgency bubbles up, like the magic porridge in danger of spilling over the edges of the cauldron, flooding the hall with a gooey mess and seeping out into the streets outside the room. The other energy is flat and still. I don't want to drown you in porridge. I don't want to pull you down into the darkness of this flatness. The mat seems roomy enough to be in all those places at once.

Witnessing

The naked branches of the trees outside the windows catch the dancer's eye. Small details shift through her

DOI: 10.4324/9781003222484-17

joints, bending cautiously, curving and straightening, twisting to the right and slightly upwards. Shifting diagonally to the left and tilting slowly, very slightly downwards. Movement supersedes thought. Gravity begins to speak. Balance whispers '…go on: it might be fun…'. The wooden surface of the floor calls the body into conversation. Impulse and impetus finds a way to spin and recover. The trees call time, reminding the world of an enduring stillness as they wait patiently for their summer leaves.

The portrait of the matriarch hanging on the wall looks on, immortalised in her youthful self, seemingly neutral, or perhaps just frightfully good at hiding her response. The mollusc senses the drama from her rockpool.

'Next!' Shouts the matriarch.

A woman tells her story as she paces emphatically, carving a figure-of-eight pathway into infinity. Is that OK? It was all about the weather. And having weathered the weather, a dance finds its way through the clouds.

A snake wriggles free of its skin.

The clock calls time.

Dropping deeper into the process

They move simultaneously on the wooden floor. Individual movement that senses another in its orbit. One foot lifts tentatively from the floor, descending with care and sensitivity, to find stability in the solid base of the floor. Sweeping my arms up, I sense my verticality, momentarily struggling with a conflict between the desire to remain still and the desire to swing my arms and move across the room. I do neither. A pheasant calls from a nearby garden and the cormorant who sits on the cliff-top returns to dance with me; the primeval shape of those drooping wings and an alertness to the other leads the way. The other human body in the room is still.

The matriarch looks on. The mollusc senses a ripple in the surface tension. The loyal soldier raises her arm, protecting matriarch, mollusc and country, or so she thinks. The snake contemplates her new skin; again. The pheasant pecks at the ground.

Onwards, upwards, downwards, backwards, in-wards and out-wards; exploring continued becomings.

Moving rocks and water

Cormorants stretch their wings on the cliffs high above. Two small birds fly down, tumbling around each other in the air and then swooping up onto a cliff ledge. Trying to run, my momentum is arrested; the weight of each step sending my feet sliding down into the shingle. The white rocks tower above me. Leaning against the side of a rock, I gaze into the ocean, beyond the horizon and into the clouds. I feel the hardness of the rock against the back of my skull. I turn to the cliff face and stretch out my left arm, flattening myself against the verticality of the surface, breathing in the smell of the chalky rock. My feet sink into the pebbles. The jagged surface of the rock face is uncomfortable and inflexible. I twist my legs and prize my feet out of the pebbles, turning to look out towards the ocean again.

The cave draws my mind's eye into a dark and secret space; enticing, mysterious and ominous. I begin to run up the beach, my speed arrested by the shingle. As each foot comes crashing into contact with the ground, the pebbles shift away from my foothold and re-position with a clatter. I shore up my energy to propel myself into the next step in a conscious act of bargaining with gravity. Each step sends a deafening roar ricocheting up my spine and into my skull. Rock and bone as one. I pause at the cave, wondering about this mysterious hollow. At the top of the cliff a cormorant opens its wings, drying her black feathers in the wind.

I stretch my arms out from my shoulders and let them droop at the joints like the cormorant. Holding the position from my shoulder blades, I swing my upper torso from left to right, dropping down onto the pebbles and I begin to roll downhill, feeling the pebbles shift beneath my body. Reaching a rock, I push myself to a standing position and climb onto its surface. The geometric shapes of the rocks around me catch my eye and my body explores the angles of one rock against another and of faults in the rocks that cause a change of tangent.

And all the time the sea comes slowly in, urging us back to base before getting cut off by the tide.

> I have a clear need to be in the liminal spaces where sea and rocks meet, among the seaweed festooned rocks,

clambering and wading in the surging channels, drawn deeper and deeper, finding (and losing) my footing blind, till it's too much and I reach for a rock with the waves coming in only to find its jagged surfaces and dark slippery strands of kelp do not make it a friendly host. I stretch out for another with the sea flooding my rolled up waterproofs so I am carrying around, then sitting in my own personal sea puddle until the sea pours out of my trouser legs. Easy to see the experience as a metaphor for my current life circumstances.

Lying on my back on rock, creature like in the bright green weed, all four limbs waving in the air I see the cracks fracturing the cliff-face from this perspective and recognise that one day the whole edifice will come tumbling down...... but not today, not today, not today...?

Two cliff-top cormorants, one white breasted, witness unperturbed. Do they recognise me as part of their world?

Later bare legged climbing and clinging over the rocks around the headland, in and out of hidden pools and crevices and the advancing tide, I morph into a long legged insect like creature both primordial and a sci-fi fantasy, relishing the pure pleasure of stretching and flexing my long jointed limbs, experiencing the world in close up, head-down, at sea-level, from ground up. I *know* this body, I *know* this terrain, I live here. Do you want to come into my lair?

Aware of your hidden presence further down the shore-line I finally spy you and stretch out an arm, with your responding raised arm I land back in my human body, taking time to re-orientate before we meet and move through the archway into the sun to where my clothes are spread-eagled, as I was earlier on the cliff–face, and lunch.

I drop to the ground and feel the pebbles pressing into my back. I don't know where she is. I allow my gaze to follow the vertical contour of the cliff face until I reach the blue sky. I open my arms to the side and imagine I have fallen from the cliff edge. In my mind's eye I trace the shape of my human body lying here. I roll my head to one side and glimpse Helen crouched by a rock with her right arm extended forwards. Does she know I'm here? I begin to roll, slowly down towards the sea. The crunching sound of the pebbles is all consuming as the ground shifts beneath my weight. I turn back to where I remember Helen had been crouching. She isn't there.

We seek each other out and shift into a collaborative movement space of companionship, finding a way to come together, two human bodies meeting with each other as well as with the materiality of the land.

We move in and out of each other's dreams.

Entanglements – back in the hall

We move in parallel, we move in relationship. We riff, embodying images and themes introduced by the other, embellishing them and handing them back. No obligation, no requirements, we are always free to leave and go our own way.

Rampaging I throw my weight around, you are unharmed. I learn that you have a different type of strength. We cross paths and swords. You are always incontrovertibly yourself. It's such a relief not to have to watch my ps and qs, untrammelled, cavorting, singing, playing, chanting,

Wild girls, unruly women, aging dancers from 2 to 102 inhabit our bodies and the space.

Trump makes an appearance and is swiftly shot down. Refugees stream through.

Border guards and soldiers strut and stride, pointing and commanding. You elude their grasp, claiming your right to occupy space.

I am at the border. In a cell. Backed up against a wall.

You are under the piano.

We're in a playground, the wild west, an audition, a dance class.

Words flood my brain, I practise discerning what is essential and let the chatter fall away.

The queen looks on, impassive, never ageing. Is she holding the space? Can she be trusted?

Through the windows trees, lambs and washing on the
line.

It's time to land again in the here and now knowing we'll
never return to this moment in time but planning to re-visit
this protected realm where no holes are barred, allowing
us to breathe, to expand, to claim time and space, to
express and replenish ourselves.

Then – nothing – as the halls lock their doors and we are
prohibited from meeting.

You disappear into your greenhouse and your Phd
as I tramp the hills.

Interrupted!

During our time of working together, and in particular the
timing of writing this article, the world became interrupted
by the Covid-19 pandemic entering the global stage. We
(humans) were stopped in our tracks and the significance
of our shared material space was amplified. This turbulent
context restricted the meeting of bodies, particularly
indoors, impacting on the studio space time that had
become an important part of our work together.

Continuing restrictions, constantly adapting to the
changing situation while trying to keep my practice afloat
and continuing to offer what I can: now meeting for
individual sessions on the beach, now offering workshops
for 6 people entirely in the landscape. Continual
cancelling, re-scheduling and re-booking depending on
how each of the halls I work in are interpreting the
guidelines, when they feel prepared to re-open and
whether they are responding to my calls or not. Writing
repeated letters detailing new arrangements, dates and
protocols. Lying awake at night. Reams of regulations,
confusing news bulletins, incompetent and coercive
government.

We compromise our schedule by spending the whole day
outside, restrictions permitting. On preparing for these all-
day-out-door meetings I realise that in this pandemic I
have spent a lot of time alone. On setting out, I find myself
becoming a little nervous of meeting with another. All my
work has moved online and I have become unfamiliar with
the journeying that characterised arrivals and departures.

I remember how, pre-pandemic, I enjoyed the journey to my own supervision, walking 40 minutes there and 40 minutes back and all that happens in that in-between space.

Setting out

I make my lunch and wander up to the greenhouse. I notice a reluctance to leave this garden. Indoors, I unzip my rucksack and reach for the items lined up on the table. Diary, notebook, pencil case, glasses, phone, tissues, sun cream, anti-bacterial hand sanitiser, face mask, bottle of cold water, flask of hot water, biodegradable teabags, lunch box with avocado, salad and fruit, woolly hat, gloves. I put my fleece, raincoat and waterproof trousers by the front door. I am in good time. Finding the keys in the glazed clay pot on the bookshelf, I step outside to be greeted by a fresh breeze on my skin, noisy rooks in the trees across the road and the smell of last night's rain.

Starting the engine, I cautiously back out of my driveway. A bird flies in front of the car and then another, dipping across the road from one hedgerow to another. I come to a passing place. The van coming towards me backs up to provide some space. I lift my hand in gratitude and edge my way past on the narrow country road.

Arrival

I arrive in our outdoor space early and spend some time acclimatising myself to the potential of this place. Helen arrives. I see her park the car from a distance. The day oozes potential. The rocks ooze potential. The earth oozes potential and far across Dartmoor, in this hazy light, I can see the sea. A small flying machine hovers in the sky. A man, with a dog on a lead, walks purposely past. We exchange a glance and a nod. I find myself arriving in the middle of an already happening world.

> It feels too long since we were able to meet. I feel the relief of not having to do anything, not having to prepare, not having to hold anything or produce anything or even to be responsible. The yearned for possibility of meeting with a friend and colleague, to breathe, to speak, to exchange and to meet the earth, rock and wind on the moor. There is a disconcerting sense of the moor as

foreign territory despite returning to this familiar tor, after four days of working intensively in coastal and woodland environments closer to home. As I see the mica glinting in the sun it's as if I don't know these rocks. Then as we open to practising in a shared vicinity I have a sense of arriving more, of the rock being both ancient and impervious, of all the thousands of years and generations of human habitation it has witnessed. It is still here, it isn't concerned about our human dramas and follies or whether we destroy ourselves, it would expect no better.

Into the woods

Prohibited from meeting inside we agree to meet on a coastal and a woodland site on the same day. There's something liberating about breaking our usual pattern. Such a relief too to be able to talk honestly about what has been happening in my life during lockdown. I have the sense I don't have to pressurise myself in any way during the session and give myself complete permission, spending time simply lying on my belly on the sloping earth as on a mother's belly.

Towards the end of the day we agree to open up to working more as a duo among the trees. I am moving between a pair of beech trees facing you working between two oaks some distance away. The oak trees are darker than the beech, their branches more crooked with frond-like upper branches, the beech trees are smoother and lighter. Playfully I celebrate that I have two arms and two legs. I pile up and move in a soft bed of leaves. I want to attract your attention and feel the impulse to disrupt what you are doing. I walk backwards towards your trees. You have made a cross of leaves and sticks between them. Thinking you were acknowledging the four directions I am shocked by the unexpected resonances with my Catholic upbringing. Elsewhere some-one has placed a wooden memorial cross in a tree. I circle one of the trees. There's a mound close-by where I once made a shrine in commemoration of my mother's death which you also imagine as a burial site. I hang from the branches of the tree wanting to go to the edge of where I can reach and lift my weight. A twig snaps. I lie in the crook of your cross and remember a shamanic burial score offered by another on this site. I feel the theme of death and am fearful I might be unwittingly invoking it but the reply comes *not yet, not yet.* Backing away from the scarred oak tree until I can really see it, reciting the Lord's prayer, I realise that I am not as scared of it as I was, the huge scar has healed and is higher up the tree, some of the wood is rotten. It is wounded but has survived, I receive this wisdom for my life. Moving away I find myself singing *As I fall on my knees with my face to the rising sun, oh Lord have mercy on me.*[1]

Later you say that the mood felt sombre and sacred.

Fragmentation – moving through

A new hall, unknown territory, neutral ground. A literal process of losing and finding each other involving stopped clocks, closed roads, lost rucksacks...
A re-entry – re-connection – re-finding our way – our way of being in the space together.... each claiming a pole, moving and speaking, entering and building on each other's images and stories, playing and responding, making free with one another's material, agreeing to each other's games... and yet a sense for me of skating over the surface... What <u>are</u> we doing, what is the intention? After moving you felt a pleasant sense of emptiness....

Washing my hands in the ladies before moving with you witnessing, I know immediately what I need to do....

Lying down on the floor to check precisely that the tape markers on the ground are <u>actually</u> 2 metres apart – unlike the miniature figures on the floor stickers which are <u>actually</u> 2 inches apart. Aware of the crucifix on the wall... *God can't help you...* and then it starts – the repetitive bouncing and shaking and chanting... **check, check, check, check**... obsessive, there's no escaping this relentless rhythm... I consent – I consent to it, knowing the personal history it refers to – I resist all the other avenues available to me in words and gesture – any temptation to theatricalise what I am experiencing, to use my training in auto-biographical performance to make this expression more digestible, more comprehensible for an audience, for others, for myself, to give it a narrative that is easier to follow. I consent to follow the pure line through, no escape... **check, check, check, check** – an authentic reflection of my internal experience, then and

now. **Check, check, check, check** – you feared you
might have to stop me – that I might go on till 7 o'clock –
check, check, check, check … still bouncing and
shaking, trapped in the rhythm… it changes to **Is it right?
Is it right? Is it right?** … on and on and on… until
without knowledge, or choice it changes again… There's
a world out there – through the windows… I continue to
follow the thread of words arising within me now moving
without speaking… The big old tree with tangly mossy
branches through the high window, gives me solace,
hope… The sky and clouds are more dangerous… I'm in
danger of dissolving. My body finds a strong physicality.
It is imperative I stay here, in my body, in the room…
strong legs, arms pointing, my movements are direct, the
form of my body clear. <u>This</u> is the antidote to the
obsessive repetition. I examine the exits, doors to
cupboards, fire exits, window sills. I do not flee but back
into a distant alcove, then sitting on the edge of the stage,
head hanging, I catch an unreadable glimpse of you…
you said it was intense, you said you couldn't find a
comfortable position from which to witness. *I didn't leave
or die, you can't expect anything more from me…*
wandering I find myself kneeling in the middle of the
room… you report a sense of sadness then reverie…

Now I <u>have</u> to look at you directly…

I wait until the moment comes… then nod and know it is
complete.

Checking out

There is such an imperative now, in this climate
emergency; this health emergency; to reconnect with the
land to locate our bodies in this space to slow down to
pause to refuse growth and to shrink. To become humble
to become smaller and to listen to these rocks that have
sat here for eons. To listen to these skylarks finding their
home. To listen to the wind as it blows across the
undulating landscape. I find I can change the way I hear
the sound of the wind by moving my head, dialoguing with
the wind, turning into it, so that it blows straight into my
face, or turning my head sideways on, to feel it on my
cheek. Moving down, I shelter behind a rock and let the
wind blow above me. Those rocks that have erupted from

the earth disrupting the smooth contours and creating interrupted flows. These meetings bring my attention to my affective and empathic capacity within an ecology of material beings. This capacity to slow down and listen moves me forwards with care.

The waves diffract, creating new patternings.

Health warning

> Our intention is to provide a window into, the flavour of, a process of peer exchange which has simply evolved over several years in this late stage of our professional lives. We are not advocating it for general consumption. These are dangerous waters to navigate safely. Sharks swim in the depths where no light penetrates, treacherous rocks threaten friendships, trauma can be re-inscribed. Self-responsibility and self-knowledge are essential, therapeutic and life experience a pre-requisite. A contained space with clear boundaries and ground rules, a degree of consciousness even in the most dynamic/charged moments, a level of trust, tried and tested, the ability for either party to step out at any point, the capacity and commitment to talk with real honesty when needed and a healthy degree of separation, are all required. With all these in place still nothing is guaranteed. Even attempting to write about it feels risky.

> We do suggest that you move with your colleagues as well as talk to them, that you have a safe creative space in which to express yourself as well as to receive and contain others. That you tailor your Continuing Professional Development to your own needs and recognise that these will be different at different stages of your (professional) life.

> Enjoy your voyaging wherever it may take you.

Note

1   This is a line from the traditional hymn (originally derived from an African American Spiritual) 'Let us break bread together on our knees' which I sang as young person.

18 Happening upon a cobweb

Caroline Frizell and Marina Rova

As we arrive into this epilogue, we are finding a way towards a transition out of this anthology and into your world. We wonder how this book will land in the world and how it will be received differently by different readers. There are multiple readings to be had by multiplicitous readers like yourself. We initially invited you into this anthology in a way that is non-linear and we wonder now, where you have arrived. As an early chapter calls us to check-in, so this epilogue is a mode of checking out.

The authors contributing to this book have offered you a commitment to nurturing and developing the role of the relational, creative moving-body-in-the-world. The interdisciplinarity and transdisciplinarity of this anthology provide a broad and unique perspective on somatic practices, integrating the crafting of practice-based processes that hold embodied creativity at their heart. The authors decolonise traditional dogma by disrupting and challenging the dualities that divide research from practice, delineate one paradigm from another and distinguish the personal from the professional, in a way that questions the performative nature of our professional roles and perspectives. This epilogue brings us into the question of how the narratives within this anthology weave patterns that offer you, the reader, the opportunity to drop into your moving body and find the creativity that is infused in every speck of dust.

In bringing this anthology to a close, we, as editors of this immediate chapter as well as the anthology, offered each other brief provocations to explore this point of transition between the doing of the editing and writing and the finalising of the manuscript before it is offered into the world. We had intended to meet in person in a studio; two bodies sharing the kinaesthetic field, generating knowledge from moving bodies. However, this was a strike period and we found ourselves meeting via zoom. We began with the question about how the contents of this anthology bring us home into the creative moving body. Marina writes:

> Starting from my belly . . . hands feeling the cloth of my top. Stroking, brushing … breathing out. Taking in my surroundings. Then this movement appeared. In and out, transferring my weight . . . shifting. Suddenly

DOI: 10.4324/9781003222484-18

my kinesphere starts to grow. This feels like (taking) a risk. Do I want to open into the field around me? Then I remembered today's date: 14th of February . . . Valentine's Day. Bleurgh! But . . . the word love arose. This book is an act of love.

And you told me you wrote down the word love before I had read it out.

Weintrobe (2021) reminds us of the importance of, and the power of love within frameworks of care, making direct links between our capacity to care and the climate chaos that has global implications. As we recall the chapters in this book, we are reminded of one of the gently pervasive thematic threads that weaves through this tapestry of chapters. That is, an impassioned plea to the readers, as practitioners, as artists, as parents and as homo-sapiens, to bring attention to the embodied experience of empathic connection with the world around us. Each of the authors brings the reader home to the creative, moving body through which we develop this relational connectivity. The book explores different ways of noticing our relational movement-based entanglements with the world around us and with each other. The tensions and contradictions that are entangled in these inquiries come to life through the creative moving body. This anthology itself invites you to pick up the torch and develop the ideas in ways that are yet unknown. Come join us in the making and the doing of this stuff. The life. The love. Part of the world's becoming in the creative immersion of embodied performance (aka life).

To decolonise our embodied practice, whether as performance artists, somatic practitioners or therapists, it is essential that we engage with critical theories that help us to question the parameters around our practices and the power imbalances that are inherent in our ontological and epistemological starting points. As practitioners, we must commit to developing anti-oppressive language and practice that challenges historical oppressions that are infused into the intersections of individual subjectivities. These include, for example, issues of gender, sexual identity, race, ethnicity, disability, class religious and spiritual beliefs, age and anthropocentrism. We must also recognise the incompleteness of the task. We may seek to understand through multiple perspectives but there will always be (some) voices that remain unheard. And we must remain alert to this at all times.

In the process of unveiling the content of this chapter, we created our movement spaces in front of the screen and moved together for ten minutes, before putting some words and images down on paper. We took turns to read out what we had written, while the other person offered their responses and thoughts as they emerged in the moment. Marina continues:

In the movement I found myself bringing my hands together as if holding a gift . . . much like the idea of making offerings.

This led to a process of sharing reflections, remembering important moments in the movement, bringing external references into the conversation, reading a quotation, noticing, making connections and linking all this back to co-authoring this epilogue. We were creating our own compass to navigate this writing. Artist, poet and performer Kae Tempest (2020) reminds us:

> The creative compass is the instinct that drew you to your discipline in the first place, and when you are in connection with it, it will tell you everything you need to know about how you are doing with your work. It will guide you through difficult creative decisions and will help you distinguish between a motivation to act from a need for approval on the one hand, and a genuine creative compulsion on the other. Sometimes the creative compass, a wounded pride and a fragile ego feel similar. They all want you to prove yourself. How do you know which is compelling you? How do you 'refind your soul'? You learn by getting it wrong.
>
> (74)

Perhaps the challenge for us, as practitioners, movers and writers, is to find ways to hold onto the creative process that continuously changes and transforms.

Caroline remembers how the timer begins. She remembers the movement experience:

> I return home to the body. I find myself standing in the centre of the room. Feet apart. Arms by my side. My arms stretch, as physical energy flows from my shoulders down into my arms to my fingers, like in one of those children's books about the human body that has a central pull out poster of the insides of the body, with nerves and tendons and muscles, bones and veins in full view. My hands reach away from me, tracing an arc in front of me across the beige carpet, towards the desk and past the laptop as I briefly glance at Marina in her virtual screen. I am confronted by the distance.

Marina too remembers a fleeting online connection in this process of simultaneous movement. She says:

> There you are, Caroline, on my screen. With me, here and far away. You reflected on the immediacy of the movement in my writing. You described it as a sensory experience, tactile. You noticed a connection between the proximity and the distance.

Our dance ends and we spend three minutes externalising our thoughts on paper. We share what we have written. We find ourselves disclosing doubts about what exactly is created, about the validity of our contribution, about the lack of time to do this epilogue justice. So be it. As we move and draw and write in our own insular spaces, disconnected from the other, we each feel safe and then as we offer our contribution into the world, we find that the marketised ideology that we smugly try to resist is actually living in us. We are reminded of our conversations with some of the authors in this anthology who grappled with the notion of self-worth, value or validity in their experience as writers. We notice that it is easier to hold on to our own value when we are disconnected. When we enter the field our value becomes diluted, or is it inadequate? There is a destructive competition in the marketisation of professional identity and practice. Do we worry so much about our image and reputation that we forget that what it is we are actually trying to do is make a connection with others and with the world around us?

We find that an intimacy is created as we share our narratives and this requires that we trust a shared ethical underpinning, i.e. that the power-relations operate with respect to anti-oppressive values at all times. No mean feat. As in social dreaming (Lawrence 2005), the deeply personal (individual dream) is offered into the public realm (the dreaming matrix) and as such, disengages from being owned by an individual and becomes part of a collective narrative. The moment of sharing in social dreaming is fragile and precarious. As the one about to share, I ask myself if I can trust the collective, if this dream (fragment) is too delicate to withstand the wider narrative and if I can bear to allow my dream to become released into the world's becoming. Caroline's dream-like exploration continues:

> Up past the window, arcing further up to the ceiling. My arms stop and there above me is a cobweb, hanging. I blow hard, the outbreath lifting my heels off the ground. The cobweb doesn't move and I'm aware that it is out of my reach. Out of the reach of my outbreath. I sense my own limitations. Another outbreath leads my body towards the ground, deflating. Another forceful outbreath lifts me again towards the cobweb on the ceiling and looking around, another cobweb catches my eye, draped around a picture-less picture rail. A shaft of sunlight enters the room through the window, illuminating the small particles of dust that are always there, floating invisibly in ever-changing patterns. My body becomes light and fluid as I become aware of being particles of dust, transient and always shifting from one state to another.

The idea of releasing these private musings, these creative writings, these intimate moments into the world makes us feel vulnerable and potentially exposed. We remember our meetings with contributing authors, who ask 'what exactly do you want?', who disclose 'I'm not sure this is good enough', who bemoan 'but there isn't time to do this justice'. There is never enough time. Marina responds to Caroline's contribution, saying:

> When I heard you read out your writing I was struck by the attention on matter, the elements, flow and space. You were surprised three minutes had gone by so quickly. There is never enough time!

If only we had more time. Deadlines become the cobweb that cannot be reached. This epilogue represents a transition from this private project that is full of imaginings and intimate musings, to a published document that is subject to the scrutiny of others. Caroline begins to move in slow motion,

> as if trying to savour the experience of this how-shall-we-do-this-epilogue dance, knowing that it is soon to come to an end. In my own world behind this screen I am free to immerse myself in whatever comes. Reaching up again, I realise that the cobweb is a distant materiality.

What is this book thing we are putting out? Perhaps it is a portal, a way into a process. We thought about the links this anthology is making with other portals into the authors' work and practice (through the images, web links, references to practice or writing) but also to the writings of other authors and practitioners who are not part of this book...branches reaching out to other areas and fields. This book does not exist in isolation. It has materialised as the paths of 16 dance, movement and somatic practitioners happened to converge to create this snapshot in this particular 21st-century moment in time. It is by no means conclusive, complete or all-encompassing, yet it is as whole as any entity in its becoming. Marina reflects on Caroline's articulation of her movement. She says:

> I was interested in the importance of breath in your movement vignette. You described happening upon a cobweb hanging from your ceiling as you reached your arms up above your head and breathed out. This seemingly simple act of having a stretch and an out-breath brought you into contact with something else . . . a cobweb. I said "don't chase the spiders away as they can warn you if there is a fire".

This animal wisdom of spiders, cats, foals and other meetings that make a difference are of an embodied nature and bring us back to the starting point for this anthology. This is our tentacular thinking (Haraway 2016) through which we sense the world, for example, via our senses, sound waves, vibrations and other forms of movement-knowledge that is beyond human language and discourse. Marina continues:

> You returned to the cobweb with intent. This time pushing the air out and reaching towards the cobweb. Exhale. To reach. . . .

There is a multiplicity of meaning in this word. As a verb, it suggests the movement of reaching out, to reach out I have to shift away from my centre... I am de-centering... Reaching also suggests an arrival...I have reached my destination. And as a noun the word reach can denote impact. This book reaches towards potential methodologies that facilitate a transformative process through the moving body, that is and was always there. The reach takes us forwards beyond our limitations, perhaps closer to things that were previously out of reach. The reach allows us to nurture the collective soil and prepare to plant seeds, the fruition of which we may never know.

To craft this epilogue, we came back to the research and practice that brings us home. Our movement explorations started from the breath and belly and moved us into the materiality of the world. This commitment to hold space for the moving relational body becomes at once the point of departure and a place of arrival to all that we know in our tacit, experiential and fleshy encounters with the world.

Whilst seeking an image for the front cover, Marina sent Caroline some paintings from her four-year-old son. Joking on WhatsApp, Marina wrote:

> "I have been looking at Yannis' art work for inspiration for the book cover:"

This was accompanied by copies of five art works. Caroline was immediately drawn to the embodied nature of the images; the shape, form, colour and the vibrant expression of the world by one small human. The images connected Caroline to her late mother, who had been a dancer and in later years an artist. With more than 90 years difference between their entrance into this world, and with the birth of one over ten years after the death of another, in Caroline's mind there was a powerful connection between Yannis's art work and that of her mother. As we moved towards finalising this transcript, mothers and sons were coming into focus. Private stories were permeating the public facing project of this writing. And as we see in the chapters that precede this epilogue, these writings bring us home to the creative moving body, and its potential to dissolve the boundaries that we create between different ways of knowing.

Caroline responded:

> "I love them. They remind me of my mother's abstract art that she painted in later years. Let's choose one".

Yannis's images interrupted our editing process in the same way that we have been calling for noticing what comes into our (kine)sphere and field of experience, how we intra-act with it and how we respond. Looking at the art work through Yannis's perspective reminds us how a connection with our creative materiality can immediately animate our life and world differently. In discussing the images with Yannis, Marina attempted an interpretation when looking at the painting entitled 'breaking the house'. Marina wondered if this was an image about constructing a house. Yannis was very direct in his response:

> "No", he said:
> "This is about breaking the house because it is so windy. The wind is blowing it away, that's why. Now there is only three (sides). That's the floor (pointing to one side) but one is missing, and one disappeared and now I have three blowing away…"

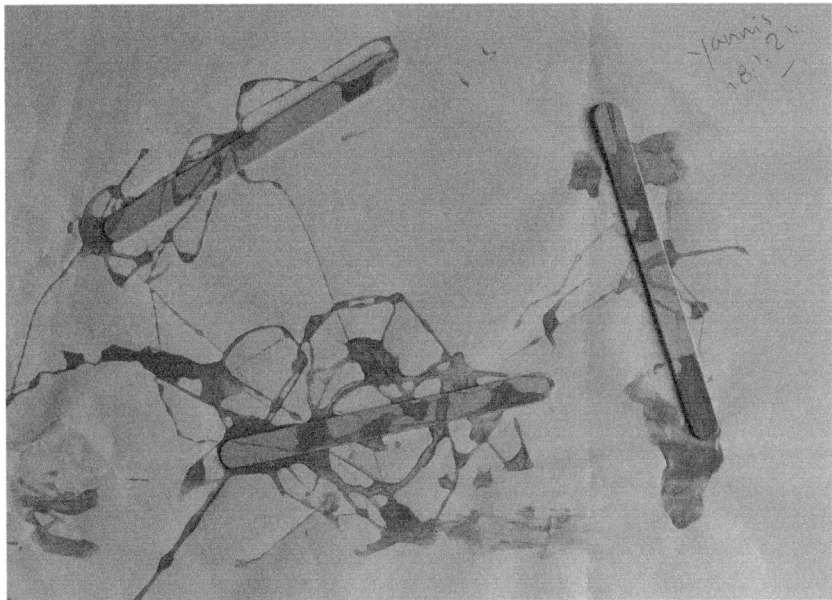

Figure 18.1 Breaking the house because it is so windy.

Yannis's conviction about the meaning of his image comes from his experiential knowledge of how it was created. He does not need sophisticated linguistic concepts to dress what he knows kinaesthetically. And the image, as a thing, is in its own right complete without the need for a representation into and/or of something else.

We leave you with Yannis's painting of the house breaking because it is so windy and this provocation to take forwards into your life (Figure 18.1):

How does your creative, moving body bring you home?

References

Haraway, D. (2016). *Staying with the trouble*. London: Duke University Press.
Lawrence, W.G. (2005). *Introduction to social dreaming: transforming thinking*. London: Karnac.
Tempest, K. (2020). *On connection*. London: Faber.
Weintrobe, S. (2021). *Psychological roots of the climate crisis*. London: Bloomsbury Press.

Index

Note: **Bold** page numbers refer to tables; *italic* page numbers refer to figures.

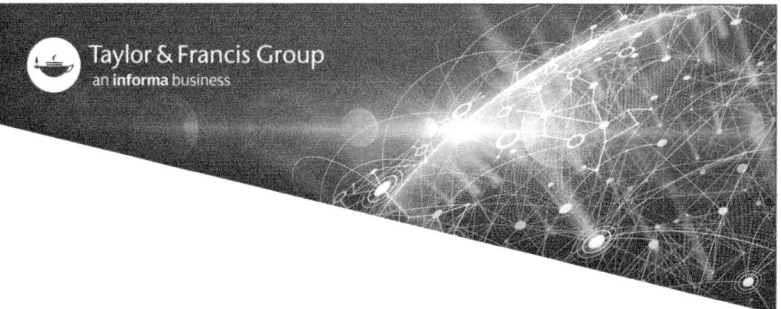
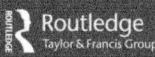
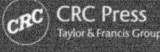